HANDBOOK OF COMMON POISONINGS IN CHILDREN
Third Edition

Author:
Committee on Injury and Poison Prevention
American Academy of Pediatrics

George C. Rodgers, Jr, MD, PhD, Editor
Nancy J. Matyunas, PharmD, Assistant Editor

American Academy of Pediatrics
PO Box 927
141 Northwest Point Blvd
Elk Grove Village, IL 60009-0927

3rd Edition
2nd Edition — 1983
1st Edition — 1978

Library of Congress Catalog Card No.: 94-71471

ISBN: 0-910761-58-2

MA0019

Quantity prices on request. Address all inquiries to:

American Academy of Pediatrics
141 Northwest Point Blvd, PO Box 927
Elk Grove Village, IL 60009-0927

The recommendations in this publication do not indicate an exclusive course of treatment or serve as a standard of medical care. Variations, taking into account individual circumstances, may be appropriate.

COMMITTEE ON INJURY AND POISON PREVENTION 1993-1994

William E. Boyle, Jr, MD, Chairperson, 1991-present
Marilyn J. Bull, MD
Murray L. Katcher, MD, PhD
S. Donald Palmer, MD
George C. Rodgers, Jr, MD, PhD
Barbara L. Smith, MD
Joseph J. Tepas, III, MD

Liaison Representatives

Jean Athey, PhD, Chief, Public Health Social Work, Maternal and Child Health Bureau

Katherine Kaufer Christoffel, MD, MPH, Ambulatory Pediatric Association

Jordan W. Finkelstein, MD, Human Learning and Behavior Branch, National Institute of Child Health and Human Development

Cheryl Neverman, Office of Occupant Protection, National Highway Traffic Safety Administration, US Department of Transportation

Richard A. Schieber, MD, Centers for Disease Control and Prevention

Milton Tenenbein, MD, Canadian Paediatric Association

AAP Section on Injury and Poison Prevention
James Griffith, MD

AAP Section on Emergency Medicine
Susan B. Tully, MD

Designated Representative
Deborah Tinsworth, US Consumer Product Safety Commission

Staff
Michelle Zajac Esquivel

ACKNOWLEDGMENTS

The Committee gratefully acknowledges the assistance of the following individuals who contributed to writing and reviewing this manual.

William Banner, Jr, MD, PhD, Primary Children's Medical Center, Salt Lake City, UT
Lorne K. Garrettson, MD, Emory University School of Medicine, Atlanta, GA
Robert J. Geller, MD, Emory University, Atlanta, GA
Frederick H. Lovejoy, Jr, MD, Children's Hospital Medical Center, Boston, MA
Ronald B. Mack, MD, Bowman Gray School of Medicine, Winston-Salem, NC
Nancy J. Matyunas, PharmD, Georgetown, IN
Howard C. Mofenson, MD, Winthrop-University Hospital, Mineola, NY
Mary Ellen Mortensen, MD, Pharmacology/Toxicology, Columbus, OH
J. Routt Reigart, MD, Medical College of South Carolina, Charleston, SC
George C. Rodgers, Jr, MD, PhD, University of Louisville, Louisville, KY
Barry H. Rumack, MD, Denver, CO
Michael W. Shannon, MD, Massachusetts Poison Control System, Boston, MA
Susan Smolinske, PharmD, Michigan Poison Center, Detroit, MI
Wayne R. Snodgrass, PhD, University of Texas Medical Branch, Galveston, TX
Milton Tenenbein, MD, Children's Hospital, Winnipeg, Canada
Sharon Vandenberg, Denver, CO

Appreciation to:

Natalie Arndt, Word Processor, Department of Maternal, Child and Adolescent Health, American Academy of Pediatrics
Barb Scotese, Senior Medical Copy Editor, Department of Maternal, Child and Adolescent Health, American Academy of Pediatrics

TABLE OF CONTENTS

INTRODUCTION

SPECIFIC POISONS

Drugs

INTRODUCTION

The *Handbook of Common Poisonings in Children* has remained over the years and through two previous editions one of the Academy's most popular and widely used publications. In 1991 the Committee on Injury and Poison Prevention reviewed the second edition originally published in 1983. It was the opinion of the Committee that 8 years of progress in the discipline of clinical toxicology made updating the handbook a necessity. This third edition is the culmination of effort by the Committee together with the assistance of Academy members with expertise in clinical toxicology.

The list of specific substances has been revised and expanded to include those drugs and chemicals commonly encountered by poison centers and other toxins that, while infrequently encountered, are commonly of concern to parents. The body of the handbook has been reorganized to group together drugs, chemical abuse agents, chemicals, and biological poisons. Generic and common chemical names have generally been used in the Table of Contents and Index, although the common trade names of some agents are included in the Index to facilitate rapid location of information.

Those familiar with the previous edition will also note some changes in the presentation of information on each toxin in an attempt to make the handbook more useful. As with previous editions, the handbook is not intended to be an exhaustive treatise. It is intended to provide the practitioner with essential information needed to assess poisoning exposures and initiate a course of action, whether that involves active intervention or only observation.

One limitation of all printed material is obsolescence. Clinical toxicology is a rapidly changing medical subspecialty and many new therapeutic approaches will occur during the lifetime of this handbook. For this reason, practitioners are strongly encouraged to consult with their local or regional poison center or medical toxicologist about all cases where significant toxicity may be expected and about toxins not found in the handbook.

EPIDEMIOLOGY OF PEDIATRIC POISONING

Accidental poisoning remains a very commonly encountered problem in children 5 years old and younger. There are no good data to indicate whether the incidence of such poisonings has decreased as a result of preventive education and such measures as child-resistant safety closures now present on many drugs and home products. There are, however, good data to substantiate a marked decline in pediatric deaths from accidental poisonings over the last 20 years. The causes for this decline certainly include the introduction of child-resistant closures and regulations governing the packaging of some medications, and may also include preventive education and improved prehospital and in-hospital care. The data compiled by the American Association of Poison Control Centers (AAPCC) Toxic Exposure Surveillance System (TESS), currently including data from 68 poison centers around the country and estimated to contain 78% of reported poisonings in the United States, documented only 152 deaths in children 5 years old and younger between 1988 and 1992.

As with younger children, data on the incidence of both accidental and intentional poisoning in older children and teenagers are also lacking. Although the number of such reported cases has steadily risen over the last decade, it is unclear if this indicates an increase in true incidence. During the same 1988 to 1992 period the AAPCC data base reported 221 deaths in children between 6 and 17 years of age. Most of these were suicides. Clearly, in terms of morbidity, this represents a much greater problem to the pediatrician. Increased use of anticipatory measures may help lower the number of such deaths.

In terms of the poisons encountered in accidental exposures, there have been few significant changes during the period covered by the AAPCC data base (1983 to 1992) and probably few major changes over the last 20 to 30 years. The common accidental exposures are to (in descending order of importance) medications, household cleaning products, personal care products such as toothpaste or cologne, and plants. The single most common cause of deaths in children 5 years old and younger is iron-containing drugs.

Most suicides or suicide gestures involve medications, either prescription or over-the-counter. The most common class of drugs responsible for deaths in the older age range are cyclic antidepressants.

POISON PREVENTION

Prevention of poisoning has always been a goal of pediatricians and the American Academy of Pediatrics. While hard data to document the effectiveness of poison prevention in reducing the incidence of poisoning are difficult to find, there is reasonable evidence to suggest that increasing parental awareness of poisoning risk will diminish the risk of mortality or serious morbidity.

It is recommended that poison prevention education begin even before a child becomes mobile. Parents should be counseled on the poisoning risks present in the home, including medications, cleaning and personal care products, plants, gardening and hobby chemicals, and other substances or items such as alcohol and cigarettes. Materials for distribution are available from the Academy as well as from most poison centers. Discussion of "poison proofing" the home by relocating toxic materials to place them out of reach; placing safety closures on cabinets, drawers, or closets containing toxic materials; and disposing of toxic and unneeded items should be part of routine counseling. Unused or outdated medications should be flushed down a toilet. Parents need to be warned that preventive measures helpful with infants and toddlers may not be adequate as children grow older. While the value of product warning stickers is controversial, parents should also be advised to discuss with children that some things are poisonous and dangerous. Parents should also be advised to keep physician and poison center numbers readily available and should be encouraged to call when an exposure or possible exposure has occurred.

Pediatricians should also be cognizant of the risk of suicide in adolescents and should discuss mental health issues with adolescent patients. If an adolescent appears depressed, the subject of suicidal ideation should be openly discussed with the patient and, if appropriate, with the parents.

OBTAINING THE HISTORY

Obtaining an accurate problem-oriented history in cases of toxic exposure is of critical importance. The following information is essential for the assessment of poisoning cases.

1. *Nature of the toxin(s):* Obtain the trade, brand, generic, or chemical name(s). It is important to be as precise as possible becaus products with very similar names may have quite different com-

positions. If the product is a mixture, concentrations or amounts of various constituents from the label are useful. Unknown product ingredients can often be identified by contacting the manufacturer. The contents of incompletely labeled prescriptions can be obtained from the dispensing pharmacy whose name and telephone number appear on the label. Prescription numbers are helpful in such cases, when available. "Unknown" tablets and capsules can frequently be identified from the imprint code on the item along with the color and shape. Parents bringing a child to the hospital or physician's office should be instructed to bring any containers involved so that information about the toxin can be confirmed.

2. *Magnitude of exposure:* In cases of ingestion, this is an estimate of the volume of liquid or the number of tablets, capsules, or other dosage forms unaccounted for. Exact quantities are rarely known, and estimates are at risk of considerable error. With liquids it is often helpful to have an adult measure the remaining volume, if any, and the original volume of the container using standard household measuring devices. It helps to remember that the average volume of a swallow in both adults and children is about 0.3 mL/kg, which can be used in some situations to estimate the volume of material consumed. In cases of intentional ingestion (suicide attempts) the history can be notoriously inaccurate, frequently grossly underestimating the amount and even the nature of what has been consumed. Patient reporting of the magnitude of exposure should be cautiously accepted and considered a minimal exposure amount. In cases of dermal, ocular, and inhalation exposures, the magnitude of exposure is assessed by estimating the concentration of the material involved and the duration of exposure.

3. *Time of exposure:* For many products, signs and symptoms of toxicity may not appear for hours or, occasionally, days following exposure. In order to assess prognosis and make therapeutic decisions, it is useful to know the time lapse between exposure and either the time of presentation or the time at which clinical abnormalities were first noted. An excellent example is acetaminophen toxicity—where treatment decisions are best made on the basis of serum levels obtained at known times after the ingestion.

4. *Progression of symptoms:* The nature and progression of signs and symptoms may be useful in determining which of several

possible toxins is actually involved in a case. The history of the progression of clinical abnormalities is often helpful in assessing both the prognosis and need for therapy. For example, a child who ingests cologne containing ethyl alcohol and is sleepy 1 hour after ingestion but becomes alert is treated differently from a child who becomes sleepy 1 hour after exposure and progressively becomes less responsive.

5. *Other medical conditions (both acute and chronic):* These problems are particularly important if the child is either taking other medications or has a medical problem, such as a seizure disorder, which may increase susceptibility to a specific toxin. It is very important with teenage girls to determine if they are pregnant. Not only is pregnancy a common precipitator of attempted suicides, but the effect of the toxin on the fetus may need to be considered.

GENERAL MANAGEMENT OF ACUTE POISONINGS

Pediatricians may encounter poisoned patients in a variety of ways. Parents often contact the pediatrician's office as a first source of information when a potentially toxic exposure occurs. This is particularly likely to occur in areas not actively served by poison centers. The problems and potential pitfalls of such telephone contact are discussed in a later section. The pediatrician may also encounter the potentially poisoned child upon presentation to the office, clinic, or an emergency department. Assessment and management of these patients are discussed in detail later. Finally, the pediatrician may be asked to see a child in consultation with possible acute or chronic poisoning. These children may present with puzzling symptoms where poisoning may be only one diagnostic consideration. It is possible to suggest a variety of toxins that might produce symptom complexes or toxidromes (see Table 7, p 34). Consultation with a regional poison center or medical toxicologist may be invaluable in these cases and may avert a slow and unnecessary workup.

DECONTAMINATION

Gastric decontamination. Preventing the absorption of ingested toxins is often a critical element in the management of the patient. Despite many years of research and experience, there is still no consensus on the optimal approach to gastric decontamination. Specific circumstances may dictate which one of the following techniques is the most appropriate. Pediatricians not experienced in the relative merits of these techniques are advised to consult with their poison center.

Emesis. The only emetic commonly used is syrup of ipecac. Syrup of ipecac contains two alkaloids with emetic activity, cephaeline and emetine. It is thought to act as both a central and local emetic. Emesis induced by syrup of ipecac only removes about a third of the gastric contents. This fact, combined with the limited toxic potential of many agents ingested by small children, mitigates against the routine use of syrup of ipecac for many childhood poisonings. For most potentially serious poisonings requiring hospital care, emesis is either contraindicated or less effective than other methods of gastric decontamination. Syrup of ipecac generally requires 20 to 30 minutes to produce vomiting and therefore has limited utility unless used soon after an ingestion (30 minutes after ingestion for liquid products and 1 to 2 hours for most solids). In some situations the ingested agent delays gastric emptying and may prolong the length of time after ingestion during which emesis is effective. The vomitus should be collected for inspection and possible analysis.

The dosage of syrup of ipecac for children 1 to 12 years of age is 15 mL, and for children >12 years of age the dosage is 30 mL. Administration of syrup of ipecac is usually followed by at least 8 ounces of water or other clear fluid. The dose can be repeated once if the initial dose fails to produce emesis within 30 minutes. For infants 6 months to 1 year, the recommended dose of syrup of ipecac is 10 mL. In this age range, however, induction of emesis should be performed under supervision, probably in a health care facility. Emesis is generally not recommended for infants under 6 months of age.

Studies have investigated the use of a single 30 mL dose of ipecac syrup in children 1 to 12 years of age. The onset of emesis was faster and the percentage of children who vomited was greater than when a 15 mL dose was administered. The side effect profile was similar for either dose. Many poison centers recommend the use of a 30 mL dose of syrup of ipecac.

Contraindications to inducing emesis include the following: altered level of consciousness, significant cardiac or respiratory symptoms, the ingestion of drugs that may produce the rapid onset of major symptoms (eg, camphor, tricyclic antidepressants), and the ingestion of caustics (acids or alkalis). Emesis is not generally recommended following the ingestion of hydrocarbons unless it is done with great care.

Syrup of ipecac may produce mild adverse effects including protracted vomiting, mild diarrhea, and transient lethargy.

Numerous studies have demonstrated that syrup of ipecac remains effective when used after its labeled expiration date. Syrup of ipecac has also been shown to be effective when the ingestant is an antiemetic.

In cases where emesis is desired and syrup of ipecac is not available, liquid dishwashing detergents (3 tablespoonfuls, or 45 mL, in a glass of water) can be safely used as an alternative. Other emetics, including salt water and finger gagging, have been shown to be unsafe, ineffective, or both and should not be used or recommended.

Gastric lavage. In older children or adults in whom large-bore (32- to 36-gauge) oral tubes can be used, gastric lavage is about as effective as emesis, removing about one third of the gastric contents. In small children in whom it is difficult to use large tubes, gastric lavage is of dubious value and generally should not be used.

The placement of oral or nasogastric tubes often precipitates gagging or emesis. For this reason the child should be positioned to minimize the risk of aspiration. Tube placement is best confirmed by the aspiration of gastric contents. If gastric contents cannot be aspirated tube placement should be confirmed by roentgenogram or the sound of bubbling upon auscultation over the stomach when air is forced through the tube.

Nasogastric or orogastric tubes generally should not be used in patients who have ingested strong acids or alkalis because the tube may perforate damaged esophageal tissue. If a tube is required, it should be placed under direct visualization using esophagoscopy. Tubes should be used with extreme care in patients who have had esophageal or gastric surgery.

Gastric contents should be aspirated and examined for the suspected poison and a sample saved for possible analysis. Lavage is then performed by instilling aliquots (15 mL/kg to a maximum of 400 mL in adolescents) of tepid isotonic saline repeated until the effluent is clear. Several liters of fluid may be required.

Activated charcoal. Activated charcoal is an effective adsorbent for many drugs and chemicals. Regular nonactivated charcoal and charcoal compressed in tablet form are ineffective as adsorbents and should not be used. Activated charcoal does not bind metals (lithium, mercury, arsenic, lead, and iron), low molecular weight alcohols (methanol and ethanol), mineral acids, alkalis, cyanide, boric acid, most organic solvents, hydrocarbons, and certain insecticides. Optimal binding is achieved with a 10:1 by weight ratio of charcoal to chemical or drug. From a practical standpoint, maximum tolerated doses are 10 to 30 g in small children and 50 to 100 g in older children and adults. Activated charcoal is available as a powder that can be made into a slurry with water or as a premixed product with or without the cathartic sorbitol. Premixed charcoal often settles out of solution and should be mixed vigorously prior to administration. Activated charcoal can usually be given orally in patients who are awake and alert. It can be flavored with cherry or coke syrup to improve acceptance. It can also be given to infants in a bottle if the nipple hole is opened slightly. Before charcoal is administered through a nasogastric or orogastric tube, tube placement *must* be confirmed by instilling some water through the tube. If any respiratory reaction occurs, the tube placement is suspect. Although direct instillation of charcoal into the lung has an ominous prognosis, aspiration of small amounts of charcoal into the lung is thought to be no worse than aspiration of gastric contents into the lung.

For many commonly encountered poisons the use of activated charcoal alone has been shown to be a more effective method of preventing absorption than either emesis or lavage. The combination of activated charcoal and gastric lavage may be the optimal method of decontamination for older children and adults. When used with lavage, activated charcoal should be given both at the beginning and at the completion of lavage.

Repeated doses of activated charcoal have been shown to increase the clearance of some toxins. It is thought that the charcoal binds toxin recycled through the gastrointestinal tract. Repeated doses should be given at 4- to 6-hour intervals usually at half of the initial dose. Do not use activated charcoal premixed with sorbitol for subsequent doses because of the risk of dehydration or electrolyte imbalance. If needed, a cathartic can be given with every fourth dose.

Activated charcoal should be administered with care in patients who have diminished or absent bowel sounds. Repeated doses of activated charcoal should not be given if bowel sounds are absent because of the risk of obstruction and aspiration.

Cathartics. There are limited data to document the efficacy of cathartics in reducing the absorption or increasing the elimination of toxins. Cathartics are generally used with activated charcoal to hasten the elimination of the toxin bound to charcoal, although there are no data that this improves the efficacy of the activated charcoal. Cathartic use is usually benign and may increase the evacuation of slowly absorbed materials, such as sustained-release products.

Sodium sulfate (Glauber salts) or magnesium sulfate (Epsom salts) is frequently used at a dose of 250 mg/kg mixed in water. Magnesium citrate solution at a dose of 4 mL/kg can also be used. Sorbitol, often supplied premixed with activated charcoal, is usually used at a dose of 1 g/kg. Repeated doses of cathartic should be used with great care because of the risk of dehydration or electrolyte imbalance.

Whole bowel irrigation. Whole bowel irrigation is the induction of a brisk fluid flow through the gastrointestinal tract using a cathartic solution, usually a mixed electrolyte or polyethylene glycol (PEG) solution such as Golytely. This technique has been used for many years to cleanse the gut prior to surgery or other procedures but has only recently found use in poisoning cases. There is limited experience in pediatric patients. It is particularly effective at removing slowly absorbed materials such as sustained-release products and slowly dissolved products such as iron tablets from the gastrointestinal tract. It has also been used to remove swallowed packets or vials of illicit drugs. The mixed electrolyte solution can be given orally or through a nasogastric or orogastric tube. The dosage is 25 to 40 mL/kg/h over 4 to 10 hours. It should be used with caution in the presence of gastric disease or ileus.

Dilution. Dilution of ingested toxins in the stomach with milk or other fluids is probably of limited value except in the case of caustic ingestion, where dilution in the oral cavity and esophagus may diminish damage. Dilution generally increases the rate of gastric emptying, which may increase the rate of absorption of some chemicals.

Skin decontamination. Dermal exposure to toxins poses two risks, absorption of the toxin through the skin and dermal injury. First remove contaminated clothing from the patient to minimize exposure. As much as 80% of the toxin is removed with clothing. Contaminated clothing should be properly discarded, particularly leather goods. Personnel decontaminating and treating the patient should wear appropriate protective apparel, including gloves. Affected skin should be cleansed with copious amounts of water or mild soap and water. Cleansing should generally be continued for 10 to 15 minutes. Avoid using abrasives because they may increase absorption by removing the stratum corneum. In the hospital, other material such as petroleum jelly, alcohol, and PEG may be used to remove specific substances not readily removed by water. Do not neutralize acids and alkalis on the skin.

Ocular decontamination. Most chemicals are only irritating to the eye. However, particularly noxious agents such as acids and alkalies are capable of rapidly causing devastating and permanent injury to the eye. For this reason, decontamination of the eye should be started as rapidly as possible. Initial decontamination involves flooding the eye with copious quantities of water, saline, or Ringer's lactate for at least 10 to 15 minutes, or longer for caustics. Avoid cold solutions because they cause discomfort. Remove contact lenses before extended flushing. Neutralization of acids and alkalis in the eye should *not* be done. Rarely, if unusual toxins are in the eye, solutions other than water may be recommended for irrigation by a poison center.

Emergency department or ophthalmologic evaluation is recommended for symptoms that persist for more than 30 minutes after rinsing, if a caustic substance is involved, or if there is any question of a foreign body sensation. Fluorescein staining or slit lamp examination may be used to detect significant damage.

Respiratory decontamination. Most acute inhalation exposures cause irritation or bronchospastic symptoms. Asphyxia or systemic toxicity may also occur. Victims should be moved to fresh air. Oxygen can be provided if the patient is experiencing respiratory difficulty.

Bronchospasm secondary to inhalation injury usually responds to inhaled bronchodilators. Symptoms resulting from the inhalation of acid fumes or chlorine may respond to inhaled dilute sodium bicarbonate solutions.

REFERRAL AND TRANSFER

The decision to transfer a poisoned patient to another facility is based on the ability of the referring physician and facility to adequately care for the patient. Considerations include the availability of special hospital resources such as laboratory support, dialysis, an intensive care unit, and the knowledge and experience of the referring physician. If resources are needed beyond the scope available locally, patients should be transferred early in the course of the poisoning when they are usually most stable.

Many exposures are unlikely to produce life-threatening symptoms or symptoms requiring specialized services. These patients can usually be most safely, conveniently, and economically treated at the initial facility or even at home. Consultation with a medical toxicologist at a poison center or poison treatment center may provide all of the information needed to treat these patients successfully. If access to more extensive laboratory testing is all that is needed, it may be easier to send samples to the laboratory rather than transfer the patient.

Before transport, poisoned patients should be maximally stabilized. This includes good intravenous access and intubation if cardiorespiratory instability is present or anticipated. Decontamination should be completed prior to transport if possible. The patient should be accompanied by staff trained to deal with any anticipated problems during transport.

TELEPHONE CONTACT

Most physicians encounter poisoning episodes first through a telephone call. When receiving a call, staff should always initially obtain the telephone number and name of the caller so contact can be reestablished if the connection is interrupted. At this point the physician or office staff person may choose to refer the caller to a local poison center. If the case is to be managed over the phone, first determine the present status of the child and attend to any life-threatening symptoms. If immediate life-saving measures are not necessary, obtain a complete history as described on pp 3-5.

With an estimate of the dose, the name of the toxin ingested, information about the present symptoms, and information about the medical history of the patient, the physician must determine the appropriate therapy. Ocular, dermal, and inhalation decontamination should be instituted at home. Emesis can be induced at home if the ingested substances and quantities can be reliably determined and emesis is the most appropriate treatment option. The child may require only observation or decontamination at home or an office visit for medical evaluation, observation, or decontamination. An emergency department visit may be required because of the potential for serious symptoms requiring medical evaluation, laboratory assessment, intensive therapy, and/or admission.

If transport to a medical facility is necessary, advise the caller about the most appropriate mode of transportation and exactly where to take the patient. If a patient is referred to a hospital, the emergency department should be advised of this referral. If syrup of ipecac is given before departure to the hospital, an attending adult must accompany the driver and patient. If convulsions, coma, or airway obstruction may develop, ambulance transport may be more appropriate. Safe driving to the medical facility should always be stressed, and the caller should be reminded to bring the drug or toxin in its container along with any vomitus.

If the patient remains at home (which occurs in about 85% of exposures), follow-up telephone contact is advised. Calls at 1, 4, and 24 hours after ingestion are appropriate in many instances. When poisoned patients are treated via telephone, a sequential record of the event should be kept (Fig 1). Every toxic ingestion should be reported to the poison center.

Poisoning Contact Form

Patient name: Date of call:

Phone number: Age:

Time of initial call: Weight:

Suspected poison: Symptoms:

History of ingestion: Recent medication use:
                                        General health:

Phone/office therapy:

Follow-up call(s) time:

Referred to hospital   Yes_____ No_____ Time_____

Referred to poison center   Yes_____ No_____ Time_____

Referred to toxicologist   Yes_____ No_____ Time_____

Outcome:

Copy of this form sent to poison control center:

Date_____

Fig 1.

LABORATORY TESTING IN POISONING

Testing for poisons or evidence of poisons in body fluids generally is the role of a hospital or reference laboratory. Although it is possible to do some qualitative testing in the office, these tests are of questionable practical value for the acute poisoning situation. While any biological sample can be analyzed, only three are routinely used in toxin assays: blood (or plasma or serum), urine, and gastric contents or aspirated gastric fluid. In general, samples of urine or gastric contents (for ingestions) are preferred for the qualitative detection of toxins. Quantitative tests should only be done on blood, plasma, or serum. Because toxin assays or screens are generally expensive, the ordering of screens on multiple samples should be discouraged unless specifically warranted.

Assays for a specific toxin or classes of toxins may be helpful in the following three ways.

1. The assay may confirm the presence of a suspected toxin or reveal an unexpected toxin.

2. A quantitative measurement of the toxin in blood may indicate whether observed symptoms are the result of that toxin or whether other causes should be investigated. For example, if a patient is thought to have ingested ethanol but the measured blood ethanol level is too low to account for the patient's symptoms, other causes should be investigated.

3. For several toxins, quantitative measurement in blood, plasma, or serum may assist in predicting the severity of exposure and the probable need for more aggressive therapy. Examples include lithium, ethylene glycol, methanol, and acetaminophen.

Drug or toxin assays are performed by a variety of techniques varying widely in their ability to detect specific agents. Most screens are capable of identifying common central nervous system active drugs such as cyclic antidepressants and commonly abused drugs such as marijuana. They may detect volatile materials such as alcohols but generally do not detect metals (including lithium), digitalis glycosides, antibiotics, some illicit drugs such as LSD or phencyclidine, and designer drugs. Check with the laboratory used by your hospital to learn what drugs or classes of drugs their screens will detect. The laboratory may be able to do a specific test for unusual agents you may suspect of being present. Quantitative tests detect only a few agents, however, and should not be ordered unless the utility of the result is known to the physician.

Other useful general laboratory tests include determinations for blood glucose, electrolytes, or serum osmolality, which may be abnormal in the presence of any of several toxins.

DRUGS USED IN POISONED PATIENTS

Office Formulary

Because it is unlikely that major poisonings will be managed in the office setting, there is little need for the pediatrician to stock more than a few drugs for poisoning management. Table 1 provides a suggested list of items for either the management of minor exposures or the initial treatment of symptomatic patients prior to transfer to the hospital.

Table 1.

Decontaminating Agents
Syrup of ipecac
Activated charcoal
Cathartic (magnesium sulfate
or magnesium citrate)

Treating Agents
Atropine
Diazepam for injection
Diphenhydramine for injection
Epinephrine (1:1000)
25% or 50% glucose
Naloxone
Oxygen

Antidotes

Table 2 provides a list of antidotes recommended for hospital use. Some drugs listed in this table may be necessary only for tertiary care facilities.

Table 2. Antidotes*

Antidote	Use	Dose	Route	Adverse Effects/ Warnings†
N-Acetylcysteine (NAC, Mucomyst)	Acetaminophen, carbon tetrachloride (experimental) and chloroform (experimental)	140/mg/kg loading, followed by 70 mg/kg every 4 h for 17 doses	PO	Nausea, vomiting
Antivenin, Crotalidae polyvalent	Rattlesnake, copperhead, and water moccasin envenomation	Dependent on weight and severity, generally 2-8 vials for initial dose	IV	Anaphylaxis is common, and serum sickness occurs in more than 75% of patients
Antivenin, *Latrodectus mactans*	Black widow spider bite	Generally one vial	IV	Anaphylaxis and serum sickness are common
Antivenin, *Micrurus fulvius*	Coral snake envenomations (eastern United States or Texas only)	Generally 4-10 vials, depends on severity	IV	Anaphylaxis and serum sickness are common
Atropine	Organophosphate and carbamate pesticides; bradycardia due to atrioventricular conduction defects	0.05 mg/kg repeated every 5-10 min as needed. Dilute in 1-2 mL of NS for ET instillation	IV/ET	Tachycardia, dry mouth, blurred vision, and urinary retention
BAL in oil (dimercaprol)	Chelating agent for arsenic, mercury, lead, antimony, bismuth, chromium, copper, gold, nickel, tungsten, and zinc	3-5 mg/kg every 4 h usually for 5-10 d	Deep IM	Local injection site pain and sterile abscess, nausea, vomiting, fever, salivation, hypertension, and nephrotoxicity (alkalinize urine)
Benztropine (Cogentin)	Acute dystonic reactions	0.02 mg/kg (1 mg max)	IV/PO	Sedation, blurred vision, dry mouth, and tachycardia

Antidote	Indication	Dose	Route	Adverse Effects
Botulinum antitoxin (from the Centers for Disease Control and Prevention through State Health Departments)	Clinical botulism	1-2 vials every 4 h for 4-5 doses	IV	Anaphylaxis, serum sickness
Cyanide antidote kit	Cyanide Hydrogen sulfide (nitrites only)	Amyl nitrite: 1 crushable ampule	Inhalation	Methemoglobinemia
		Sodium nitrite: 0.33 mL/kg of 3% solution if hemoglobin level not known, otherwise based on tables with product	IV	Methemoglobinemia
		Sodium thiosulfate: 1.6 mL (400 mg)/kg of 25% solution, may be repeated every 30-60 min to a maximum of 50 mL	IV	
Deferoxamine (Desferal)	Iron	Infusion of 15 mg/kg/h (max 6 g/d)	IV (preferred)	Hypotension (minimized by avoiding rapid infusion rates)
		IM: 1 g load, then 0.5 g every 4 h	IM	

Table 2. Antidotes* *(continued)*

Antidote	Use	Dose	Route	Adverse Effects/ Warnings†
Digoxin-specific Fab antibodies (Digibind)	Digitalis glycosides (synthetic or natural)	One vial binds 0.6 mg of digitalis glycoside; ingested dose may be estimated from serum level (see table with product)	IV	Allergic reactions (rare), return of condition being treated with digitalis glycoside
Diphenhydramine (Benadryl)	Extrapyramidal symptoms, acute dystonic reactions, allergic reactions	0.5-1 mg/kg every 4-8 h 300 mg/24 h max	IV/PO	Sedation or paradoxical agitation, ataxia
Dimercaptosuccinic acid (succimer, DMSA, Chemet)	Lead, and probably mercury, arsenic, and perhaps other metals	10 mg/kg every 8 h for 5 d, then 10 mg/kg every 12 h for 14 d	PO	Nausea and vomiting
EDTA, calcium	Lead, manganese, nickel, zinc, and perhaps chromium	1-1.5 g/m²/d in divided dosages every 4-12 h for 5 d	IM	Nausea, vomiting, fever, hypertension, arthralgias and allergic reactions, local inflammation, and nephrotoxicity (maintain adequate hydration)
Ethanol (ethyl alcohol)	Methanol, ethylene glycol	750 mg/kg loading dose followed by 100-150 mg/kg/h infusion of 5% or 10% ethanol	IV/PO	Nausea, vomiting, sedation

Drug	Dose	Route	Side Effects/Notes
Flumazenil (Romazicon)	0.3 mg every 1 min to a max of 3 mg	IV	Nausea, vomiting, facial flushing, agitation, headache, dizziness, seizures. Do not use for unknown or antidepressant ingestions. **NOTE: May not reverse respiratory depression.**
Benzodiazepines			
Folic acid (Folvite)	1 mg/kg every 4 h	IV	Uncommon
Methanol			
Ethylene glycol (investigational)			
Glucagon	0.15 mg/kg bolus followed by infusion of 0.05-0.1 mg/kg/h	IV	Hyperglycemia, nausea, and vomiting
β-blockers, calcium channel blockers, hypoglycemic agents			
Hydroxocobalamin (Vitamin B_{12a})	50 times the amount of cyanide	IV	**NOTE: Not presently available in the United States for this indication.**
Cyanide (investigational)			
Methylene blue	0.1-0.2 mL/kg of 1% solution, slow infusion, may be repeated every 30-60 min	IV	Nausea, vomiting, headache, dizziness
Methemoglobinemia			
Naloxone (Narcan)	0.01 mg/kg; if no effect, give 0.1 mg/kg; may be repeated as needed; may give continuous infusion	IV	Acute withdrawal symptoms if given to addicted patients
Narcotics Clonidine (inconsistent response)			
d-Penicillamine (Cuprimine)	25-100 mg/kg/d divided four times a day (max 1 g)	PO	Allergic reactions, anorexia, nausea, and vomiting
Chelating agent for lead, mercury, arsenic, and copper			

Table 2. Antidotes* *(continued)*

Antidote	Use	Dose	Route	Adverse Effects/Warnings†
Physostigmine (Antilirium)	Anticholinergic agents	0.02 mg/kg; slow push	IV	Bradycardia, asystole, seizures, bronchospasm, vomiting, headache. **NOTE: Do not use for cyclic antidepressants.**
Pralidoxime (2-PAM, Protopam)	Organophosphates	25-50 mg/kg over 5-10 min (max 200 mg/min), can be repeated every 1 h as needed	IV	Nausea, dizziness, headache. Tachycardia, muscle rigidity, and bronchospasm (rapid administration)
Pyridoxine (Vitamin B₆)	Isoniazid, *Gyromitra* mushrooms Ethylene glycol (investigational)	Isoniazid: dose = dose of isoniazid ingested mushrooms: 25 mg/kg ethylene glycol: 50 mg/kg	IV	Uncommon
Vitamin K (Aqua Mephyton)	Coumadin, indanedione rodenticides	1-5 mg repeated every 6-8 h as needed	SC or IM	Uncommon

*Only general indications and contraindications are given. For serious poisonings, particularly with multiple agents, consult a toxicologist or other specialist to ascertain which treatment regimens may be appropriate. PO indicates orally; IV, intravenously; SC, subcutaneously; IM, intramuscularly; SL, sublingually; ET, endotracheal tube.
†History of sensitivity to a drug is always a contraindication.

Other Drugs Useful for Poisonings

Table 3 lists other drugs commonly used in the treatment of pediatric poisoning. Only general indications and contraindications are given. For serious poisonings, particularly with multiple agents, consult a medical toxicologist or other specialist to ascertain which treatment regimens may be appropriate.

Table 3. Other Drugs Useful for Treating the Poisoned Patient*

Drug	Indication(s)	Dose	Route	Adverse Effects	Contraindications†
Activated charcoal	Adsorbent	10 to 100 g (or 10 times the weight of ingested material)	PO	Vomiting, intestinal obstruction (rare), aspiration pneumonia	Caustics, absent bowel sounds
Bicarbonate, sodium	Metabolic acidosis, or for alkaline diuresis (salicylate, phenobarbital)	0.5-1 mg/kg, repeat as needed	IV	Hypernatremia, metabolic alkalosis	Hypernatremia
Bretylium (Bretylol)	Ventricular fibrillation	5 mg/kg over 1 min. Repeat every 10-20 min to 30 mg/kg max	IV	Hypotension, vomiting	Use with caution in cyclic antidepressant and digitalis glycoside intoxication
Calcium chloride (10%)	Hypocalcemia, calcium channel blockers	0.1-0.2 mL/kg slow push every 10 min	IV	Tissue irritation, hypotension, dysrhythmias from rapid injection	Digitalis glycoside intoxication
Calcium gluconate (10%)	Hypocalcemia, fluoride, calcium channel blockers, hydrofluoric acid	0.2-0.3 mL/kg slow push; repeat as needed For hydrofluoric acid burns topical gel (1 g in 30 g water-soluble base) or intradermal (0.5-1 mL/cm² affected skin)	IV	Tissue irritation, hypotension, dysrhythmias from rapid injection	Digitalis glycoside intoxication

Drug	Indication	Dose	Route		
Dantrolene (Dantrium)	Malignant hyperthermia	1 mg/kg every 10 min to max 10 mg/kg, then switch to oral administration 4-8 mg/kg/24 h PO divided 4 times a day for 3-4 d	IV	Muscle weakness	None
Diazepam (Valium)	Seizures, anxiety reaction	0.1-0.2 mg/kg, repeat as needed	IV	Respiratory depression, central nervous system depression	None
Diazoxide (Hyperstat)	Hypertensive crisis Oral hypoglycemic ingestion	1-3 mg/kg (150 mg max) every 5-15 min 3-5 mg/kg (300 mg max) every 6 h	IV	Hypotension, hyperglycemia	Hypertension due to cardiac or vascular malformation
Dobutamine (Dobutrex)	Hypotension of cardiac origin	2.5-15 µg/kg/min to 40 µg/kg/min max	IV	Tachycardia, dysrhythmias, hypertension	Hypertension
Dopamine (Intropin)	Hypotension	2-20 µg/kg/min	IV	Hypertension, dysrhythmias, extravasation injury	Hypertension, avoid in hydrocarbon exposures

Table 3. Other Drugs Useful for Treating the Poisoned Patient* *(continued)*

Drug	Indication(s)	Dose	Route	Adverse Effects	Contraindications†
Epinephrine (1:10 000)	Cardiac arrest, hypotension	0.1 mL/kg every 3-5 min or 0.1-1.0 µg/kg/min infusion	IV	Tremor, headache, hypertension, dysrhythmias	Hypertension, avoid in hydrocarbon exposures
(1:1000) (Adrenalin)	Allergic reactions, anaphylaxis	0.01 mL/kg/dose (0.3 mL max) every 15 min (4 doses max or every 4 h as needed)	SC or ET		
Esmolol (Brevibloc)	Tachydysrhythmias, hypertension	50-100 µg/kg/min infusion	IV	Hypotension, bradycardia, bronchospasm	Asthma, use with caution in presence of cardio-depressant drugs
Haloperidol (Haldol)	Agitation and acute psychosis	0.01-0.15 mg/kg/24 h divided every 8 h	IM or PO	Respiratory depression, anticholinergic symptoms, decreased seizure threshold, extrapyramidal symptoms	Central nervous system depression

Drug	Indication	Dose	Route	Adverse effects	Contraindications
Ipecac syrup	Emesis	Age 6 mo-1 y: 10 mL Age 1-12 y: 15 mL >12 y: 30 mL May repeat once if no emesis in 30 min	PO	Lethargy, persistent vomiting, diarrhea	Decreased level of consciousness, likelihood of development of major symptoms, caustics, hydrocarbons
Isoproterenol (Isuprel)	Bradycardia	0.1-1.0 µg/kg/min infusion	IV	Myocardial anoxia, ventricular dysrhythmia, hypotension	Avoid in hydrocarbon exposure, ventricular fibrillation, or tachycardia (except for torsade de pointes)
Labetalol (Normodyne)	Hypertension with tachycardia	0.25 mg/kg push over 2 min	IV	Hypotension or hypertension, bronchospasm, nausea, and diarrhea	Asthma, congestive heart failure
Lidocaine (Xylocaine)	Ventricular dysrhythmias	1 mg/kg as bolus over 1 min followed by an infusion 20-50 µg/kg/min	IV ET (bolus dose only)	Dizziness and drowsiness, nausea, flushing	Epilepsy
Lorazepam (Ativan)	Seizures, anxiety	0.1 mg/kg/dose to 4 mg/dose max	IV	Respiratory and central nervous system depression	None
Methocarbamol (Robaxin)	Muscle spasms from black widow spider and strychnine	15 mg/kg over 5 min, then 10 mg/kg over 4 h	IV	Dizziness, drowsiness, nausea, flushed skin	Epilepsy

Table 3. Other Drugs Useful for Treating the Poisoned Patient* *(continued)*

Drug	Indication(s)	Dose	Route	Adverse Effects	Contraindications†
Metoclopramide (Reglan)	Nausea and vomiting	1-2 mg/kg over 15 min every 2-6 h	IV	Sedation, extrapyramidal symptoms	Epilepsy
Midazolam (Versed)	Seizures, anxiety	0.05-0.1 mg/kg (0.2 mg/kg IM), repeated as needed	IV/IM	Respiratory depression	None
Nifedipine (Procardia)	Severe hypertension	0.25-0.5 mg/kg/dose repeat every 6-8 h as needed	PO/SL	Hypotension, tachycardia, headache	None
Nitroprusside (Nipride)	Severe hypertension	0.5-10 µg/kg/min as a continuous infusion, titrated to effect	IV	Hypotension, nausea, vomiting, headache, cyanide toxicity	Use with care in renal failure
Norepinephrine (Levophed)	Shock with hypotension	Begin infusion at 0.1 µg/kg/min and increase every 5-10 min until desired effect	IV	Hypertension	Hypertension. Avoid in hydrocarbon exposure
Phenobarbital (Luminal)	Seizures	10-15 mg/kg loading dose, slow infusion	IV	Respiratory and central nervous system depression	None

Drug	Indications	Dose	Route	Side effects	Contraindications
Phentolamine (Regitine)	Hypertensive crisis, extravasation of vasoconstrictors	0.02-0.1 mg/kg as a bolus or 0.1-0.2 mg/kg diluted and injected into area of extravasation	IV	Hypotension, tachycardia	None
Phenytoin (Dilantin)	Seizures, cardiac dysrhythmias	15-20 mg/kg load, 5 mg/kg/d maintenance	IV/PO	Hypotension	Heart block, infuse no faster than 50 mg/min
Propranolol (Inderal)	Sinus tachycardia, ventricular dysrhythmias, thyroid hormone intoxication	0.01 mg/kg/dose IV (max 1 mg) every 6-8 h or 0.5-4 mg/kg/d PO divided every 6 h	IV/PO	Bradycardia, hypotension, bronchospasm	Asthma; use with caution in the presence of cardiac depressant drugs
Sodium polystyrene sulfonate (Kayexalate)	Hyperkalemia	1 g/kg as a suspension	PO/PR	Diarrhea, hypokalemia	None

*Only general indications and contraindications are given. For serious poisonings, particularly with multiple agents, consult a toxicologist or other specialist to ascertain which treatment regimens may be appropriate. PO indicates orally; IV, intravenously; SC, subcutaneously; IM, intramuscularly; SL, sublingually; ET, endotracheal tube; PR, rectally.

†History of sensitivity to a drug is always a contraindication.

TOXICITY CALCULATIONS

The Anion Gap

The anion gap is the difference between measured serum cations and anions and represents unmeasured anions.

$$\text{Anion gap} = [Na] - ([Cl] + [HCO_3])$$

The normal range is 8 to 12 mEq/L. Toxins or diseases frequently leading to an elevated anion gap include *A*lcohol, *T*oluene, *M*ethanol, *U*remia, *D*iabetic acidosis, *P*araldehyde, *I*ron, *L*actic acid, *E*thylene glycol, *S*alicylates. Remember the mnemonic AT MUD PILES.

Reference
Oh MS, Carrol HJ. The anion gap. *N Engl J Med.* 1977;279:814

The Osmolal Gap

The osmolal gap is the difference between the measured (by freezing point depression) and the calculated serum osmolarity.

$$\text{Osmolal gap} = \text{Osm (measured)} - \text{Osm (calculated)}$$

$$\text{Osm (calculated)} = 1.86\,[Na] + \frac{[glucose]}{18} + \frac{[BUN]}{2.8}$$

The normal gap is <10 mOsm.

Toxins that produce an increased osmolal gap include alcohols (methanol, ethanol), glycols, mannitol, acetone (diabetes), chloroform, sorbitol, and paraldehyde.

Reference
Gennair FJ. Current concepts. Serum osmolality: uses and limitation. *N Engl J Med.* 1984;310:102-105

Blood Ethanol Levels

The following formula can be used to predict the peak blood ethanol level after a single ingestion by a nonalcoholic person:

$$C_p = \frac{\text{Dose}}{V_d \times \text{body weight}}$$

C_p = peak plasma concentration in mg/L

Dose = milligrams of ethanol ingested

V_d = volume of distribution of ethanol in liters per kilogram body weight

V_d (adult) = 0.6 L/kg

V_d (child) = 0.7 L/kg

Body weight = weight of patient in kilograms

The specific gravity of alcohol (ETOH) is 0.790, therefore 1 mL 100% ETOH = 790 mg

See Ethanol (Ethyl Alcohol) (p 149) for the alcohol content of beverages and other products.

Example:
A 20-kg child drinks 10 mL of perfume with an alcohol content of 80% (v/v). What peak alcohol level would be expected?

$$C_p = \frac{\text{Dose}}{V_d \times \text{body weight}}$$

Dose (mg) = volume ingested (mL) x % ethanol x specific gravity x 1000

Dose (mg) = 10 mL x 0.80 x 0.79 x 1000

Dose = 6300 mg

$$C_p = \frac{6300 \text{ mg}}{0.7 \text{ L/kg} \times 20 \text{ kg}}$$

C_p = 450 mg/L = 45 mg/dL (mg%)

The same formula can suggest the dose of ethyl alcohol needed to achieve a given blood ethanol level to treat methyl alcohol or ethylene glycol intoxications.

Example:

To achieve an ethanol level of 100 mg/dL (1000 mg/L) in a 20-kg child, how many milliliters of absolute (100%) ethanol must be used?

Dose (mg) = C_p x V_d (L/kg) x body weight (kg)

Dose (mg) = 1000 mg/L x 0.7 L/kg x 20 kg

Dose = 14 000 mg, or 14 g

$$\text{Dose in milliliters of 100\% ethanol} = \frac{\text{Dose in grams}}{\text{specific gravity}}$$

$$\text{Dose (mL of 100\% ethanol)} = \frac{14}{0.79} = 17.7 \text{ mL}$$

Ethanol is metabolized at the rate of approximately 125 mg/kg/h in a nonalcohol-dependent person with normal liver function. To maintain a specific blood ethanol level after the loading dose, an infusion rate of approximately 125 mg/kg/h is needed. **The first maintenance dose should be given concurrent with the loading dose.** If dialysis is instituted, the infusion rate of ethanol requires adjustment.

Another approach for calculating doses for ethanol therapy uses:

10% w/v ethanol in D_5W for intravenous administration.

Loading dose: adult, 7.5 mL/kg; child, 8.75 mL/kg.
Maintenance dose: adult, 1.25 mL/kg/h; child, 1.25 mL/kg/h.

Infuse both the loading dose and the first hourly dose over the first hour. Check blood alcohol level after 2 hours. The goal is to achieve and maintain a level of 100 to 150 mg/dL. Dialysis increases the required dose by a variable amount, depending on the efficiency of the dialysis system. These are initial doses. Great variation between patients requires individualization of the ethanol dose.

Reference

Harmon WE, Sargent JA. Ethanol during hemodialysis for ethylene glycol poisoning. *N Engl J Med.* 1981;305:522

NONTOXIC INGESTIONS

Many items commonly found in and around the home are essentially nontoxic when ingested in small to modest quantities (Table 4). Some of these materials may produce minor gastrointestinal symptoms (stomachache, vomiting, or diarrhea) which usually do not require treatment. Children ingesting these materials can almost always be managed at home with parental observation. If exceptionally large quantities are ingested, consultation with a poison center is advised.

Table 4. Frequently Ingested Products That Are Usually Nontoxic*

Abrasives	Iodophil disinfectants
Adhesives	Laxatives
Antacids	Lipstick
Antibiotics	Lubricating oils (unless aspirated)
Ballpoint pen inks	Magazines
Bathtub floating toys	Magic markers
Bath oil (castor oil and perfume)	Makeup
Body conditioners	Matches
Bubble bath soaps (detergents)	Mineral oil (unless aspirated)
Calamine lotion	Newspaper (chronic ingestion
Candles (beeswax or paraffin)	may result in lead poisoning)
Caps (toy pistols, potassium	Paint- indoor latex
chlorate)	Pencil lead (graphite, coloring)
Chalk (calcium carbonate)	Petroleum jelly (Vaseline)
Children's toy cosmetics	Play-Doh
Clay (modeling)	Polaroid picture coating fluid
Contraceptive agents	Porous-tip ink marking pens
Corticosteroids	Prussian blue (ferricyanide)
Cosmetics	Putty
Crayons (marked A.P. or C.P.)	Rubber cement
Dehumidifying packets (silica or	Sachets
charcoal)	Shampoo
Deodorants — under arm	Shaving creams and lotions
Etch-A-Sketch	Soap and soap products
Fabric softeners	Spackles
Fertilizers (if no insecticide or	Suntan preparations
herbicides added)	Sweetening agents (saccharin,
Fish bowl additives	aspartame)
Glues and pastes	Teething rings (may be filled with
Golf ball (core may cause mechanical	unsterile water)
injury)	Thermometers (mercury)
Grease	Toothpaste (with and without
Hand lotions and creams	fluoride)
Hydrogen peroxide (medicinal 3%)	Warfarin rodenticides (<0.5%)
Incense	Water color paints
Indelible markers	Zinc oxide
Ink (black, blue — nonpermanent)	

*Unlikely to produce more than mild symptoms unless exceptional quantities are involved or the patient is allergic to the material.

Consumption of plant parts is very common by small children. Only a few plants are capable of causing life-threatening symptoms in children; however, many plants can produce mild to moderate gastrointestinal symptoms (see section on plants, p 247). Tables 5 and 6 list some common household and garden plants and berries that are unlikely to cause toxic symptoms. Although home observation is usually adequate treatment, plant parts, including berries, may, on rare occasions, be aspirated or cause intestinal obstruction.

Table 5. Nontoxic House and Garden Plants

Abelia
African violet (*Saintpaulia ionantha*)
Airplane plant
Airplane propeller plant (*Crassula culturata*)
Aluminum plant (*Pilea cadieri*)
Aralia false (*Dizygotheca elegantissima*)
Aster (*Aster annual*)
Begonia species
Boston fern (*Nephrolepis exalata*)
Carnation (*Dianthus caryophyllus*)
Cast-iron plant (*Aspidistra elatior*)
Chinese evergreen (*Aglanonema* sp)
Christmas cactus (*Zygocactus truncatus*)
Coleus sp
Corn plant (*Dracena fragrans*)
Dahlia (*Dahlia* sp)
Daisy (*Chrysanthemum* sp)
Dandelion (*Taraxacum* sp)
Day lily (*Hemerocallis* sp)
Donkey tail (*Sedum morganianum*)
Dracaena species
Easter cactus (*Schulmbergera bridgesii*)
Fern species (except *Asparagus*)
Fig (*Ficus*)
Gardenia (*Gardenia jasminoides*)
Geranium (*Pelargonium* sp)
Hawaiian Ti (*Cordyline terminalis*)
Hen and chicks (*Astlenium bulbiferum*)
Honeysuckle (*Lonicera* sp)

Hoya (wax plant)
Impatiens (*Impatiens* sp)
Jade plant (*Crassula argentea*)
Kalanchoe (*Kalanchoe* sp)
Lipstick plant (*Aeschynanthus lobbianus*)
Magnolia (*Magnolia stellata*)
Marigold (*Tagetes* sp and *Calendula officinalis*)
Monkey plant (*Ruellia makoyana*)
Mother-in-law's tongue (*Sansevieria trifasciata*)
Nasturtium (*Trapaeloum majus*)
Norfolk Island Pine (*Araucaria heterophylla*)
Palm species
Petunia (*Petunia* sp)
Peperomia (botanical name)
Piggyback plant (*Tolmiea menziesii*)
Pilea (botanical name)
Pink polka dot plant (*Hypoestes sanguinolenta*)
Poinsettia (*Euphorbia pulcherrima*)
Prayer plant (*Marantan leuconeura, "Kerchoveana"*)
Pyracantha (*Pyracantha coccinea*)
Rose (*Rosa* sp)
Rubber plant (*Ficus elastica*; may cause dermatitis)
Schefflera (*Brassaia actinophylla*)
Sensitive plant (*Mimosa pudica*)
Snake plant (mother-in-law's tongue, *Sansevieria*)

Table 5. Nontoxic House and Garden Plants *(continued)*

Snapdragon (*Antirrhinum coulteranum*)
Spider plant (*Anthericum* or *Chlorophytum comosum*)
Strawberry, mock or Indian (*Duchesnea indica*)
Swedish ivy (*Plectranthus australis*)
Violet (*Viola* sp)

Wandering Jew (*Zebrina pendula*)
Weeping fig (*Ficus benjamina*; may cause dermatitis)
Yucca plant (*Yucca aliofolia marginata*)
Zebra plant (*Aphelandra squarrosa*)

Table 6. Nontoxic Berries

Common Name	Botanical Name	Color of Berry (Season)
Aucuba	*Aucuba japonica*	Red (autumn)
Barberry	*Berberis* species	Orange-red (autumn) Tan-spotted (winter)
Dogwood, flowering	*Cornus florida L.*	Red (August to November)
Nandina	*Nandina domestica*	Red (summer and autumn)
Highbush cranberry	*Viburnum trilobum*	Red (late summer and autumn)
Mountain ash	*Sorbus aucuparia*	Orange (later summer and autumn)
Pokeberry	*Phytolacca americana*	Purple (late summer and autumn)
Pyracantha*	*Pyracantha coccinea*	Red (late summer and autumn)

*May have poisonous varieties.

TOXIDROMES

Table 7 provides a collection of symptoms associated with certain classes of poisons: these are termed "toxidromes." Toxidromes assist in making a diagnosis in a patient when the toxin is not known. They are also useful for anticipating other symptoms that are likely to occur.

Table 7. Common Toxic Syndromes

Syndrome	Symptoms	Sources
Anticholinergic	Exocrine gland hyposecretion, thirst, flushed skin, dilated pupils, hyperthermia, urinary retention, delirium, hallucinations, tachycardia, respiratory insufficiency	Belladonna alkaloids, jimson weed, some mushrooms, antihistamines, tricyclic antidepressants, scopolamine
Cholinergic (muscarinic and nicotinic)	Exocrine gland hypersecretion, urination, gastric symptoms, muscle fasciculations, weakness or paralysis, bronchospasm, tachycardia or bradycardia, convulsions, coma	Organophosphate and carbamate insecticides, some mushrooms, tobacco, black widow spider bites (severe)
Extrapyramidal	Tremor, rigidity, opisthotonus, torticollis, dysphonia, oculogyric crisis	Phenothiazines, haloperidol, metoclopramide
Hypermetabolic	Fever, tachycardia, hyperpnea, restlessness, convulsions, metabolic acidosis	Salicylates, some phenols, triethyltin, chlorophenoxy herbicides
Narcotic	Central nervous system depression, hypothermia, hypotension, hypoventilation, small pupils	All narcotics including Lomotil, propoxyphene, and heroin
Sympathomimetic	Excitation, psychosis, convulsions, hypertension, tachypnea, hyperthermia, dilated pupils	Amphetamines, phencyclidine, cocaine and crack cocaine, phenylpropanolamine, methylphenidate, theophylline, caffeine
Withdrawal	Abdominal cramps, diarrhea, lacrimation, sweating, "goose flesh," yawning, tachycardia, restlessness, hallucinations	Cessation of intake of alcohol, barbiturates, benzodiazepines, narcotics

SPECIFIC POISONS

DRUGS

Acetaminophen

Available Forms and Sources: Acetaminophen is supplied as various solid and liquid oral dosage forms, and as rectal suppositories. It is also a component of many cold and analgesic mixtures. The exact product name must be checked for acetaminophen concentration.

Mechanism of Toxicity: Acetaminophen undergoes microsomal metabolism to a highly reactive metabolite that binds covalently to hepatic cell constituents causing hepatocellular necrosis. Young children are generally at less risk for hepatotoxicity from a given acetaminophen level than adults. It has been postulated that this difference is due to a higher glutathione turnover rate in children, which results in more rapid detoxification of acetaminophen's reactive metabolites.

Toxic Dose: A potentially acute toxic dose of acetaminophen is 150 mg/kg for children under 12 years of age, or 7.5 g for children over 12 years of age. Unique patient factors, however, may influence this. In infants and children, chronic ingestion of greater than 140 mg/kg/d for 2 to 3 days has been associated with hepatotoxicity.

Signs and Symptoms: No significant signs or symptoms occur within the first 24 hours of an acetaminophen overdose. Patients may exhibit generalized malaise, nausea, vomiting, and drowsiness between 6 and 12 hours after ingestion. A latent period of 24 to 36 hours, which may continue for up to 5 days, may occur between ingestion and onset of hepatic symptoms. Hepatotoxicity, manifested by elevated levels of liver enzymes and bilirubin, and disturbances in clotting mechanisms can be life-threatening. Metabolic acidosis, renal damage or insufficiency, myocardial damage, neurologic signs including coma, and pancreatitis also have been associated with acute severe acetaminophen toxicity.

Diagnostic Testing: Acetaminophen is detected in most routine drug screens. A plasma acetaminophen concentration should be obtained no sooner than 4 hours following the ingestion. Plot the acetaminophen concentration on the Rumack-Matthew Nomogram (Figure 2) to estimate the potential for hepatotoxicity if the patient remains untreated with the antidote. It is not necessary or helpful to obtain additional serum acetaminophen levels.

General Treatment: Significant acute symptoms are not anticipated, although hospitalization generally is required to treat significant exposures.

Decontamination: (**Refer to the treatment section p 6 for the appropriate use of these techniques.**) Emesis may be useful if instituted soon after ingestion (approximately 90 minutes). Gastric lavage may be used when appropriate. The administration of activated charcoal is suggested for patients who are initially seen within 4 hours of an acetaminophen overdose to minimize drug absorption. The preferred cathartic may be magnesium sulfate or sodium sulfate on the theory that some of the sulfate will be absorbed and reduce the toxicity of the acetaminophen.

Antidote: *N*-acetylcysteine (NAC, Mucomyst) is most effective if administered within 16 hours after ingestion. The efficacy of NAC treatment started more than 24 hours after ingestion has not been established. NAC should be administered if the plasma acetaminophen concentration is in the toxic range, or if a toxic dose (150 mg/kg, 7.5 g) is suspected to have been ingested within 24 hours of presentation and an acetaminophen plasma concentration is not readily available. Treatment with NAC is not indicated for chronic ingestions. The oral loading dose is 140 mg/kg of 10% or 20% *N*-acetylcysteine diluted to a 5% solution with water, a cola drink, or fruit juice. Follow the loading dose with 17

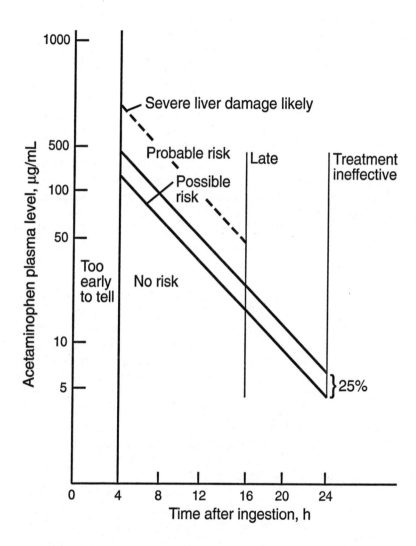

Fig 2. Treatment protocol for acetaminophen. Adapted from Rumack BH, Peterson RC, Koch GG, Amara IA. Acetaminophen overdose: 662 cases with evaluation of oral acetylcysteine treatment. *Arch Intern Med.* 1981;141:382

maintenance oral doses of 70 mg/kg, each diluted with water, a cola drink, or fruit juice given at 4-hour intervals. Do NOT discontinue NAC treatment prematurely if subsequent plasma acetaminophen levels fall below the toxic line on the nomogram. All clinical data on the efficacy of oral NAC as an antidote for acetaminophen hepatotoxicity are based on completion of all 17 maintenance doses. Repeat any dose of NAC one time if it is vomited within 1 hour of administration.

Intravenous (IV) NAC protocols have been investigated. Intravenous NAC appears to be safe and effective, and is pending approval by the Food and Drug Administration. The manufacturer recommends use of only the pyrogen-free NAC, which is not yet commercially available. A loading dose of 140 mg/kg of 0.2 g/mL of N-acetylcysteine diluted 1:5 in 5% dextrose in water is administered IV over 1 hour, followed by 12 maintenance doses of 70 mg/kg of NAC diluted 1:5 in 5% dextrose in water given at 4-hour intervals.

Specific Treatment: For ingestions of more than one substance, when multiple-dose charcoal is indicated, administer a dose of activated charcoal and cathartic and obtain a plasma acetaminophen concentration. If the concentration is potentially hepatotoxic, insert a nasogastric tube, lavage the stomach to remove any residual charcoal, and administer NAC orally. If repeated dose activated charcoal must be used, alternate charcoal and NAC doses every 2 hours, and lavage to remove any residual charcoal before each NAC dose.

If persistent vomiting develops, verify that the patient is receiving a 5% solution of NAC and not full-strength NAC. Administer the NAC dose slowly over 30 to 60 minutes via nasogastric tube. To help control vomiting, administer metoclopramide (Reglan), 1 mg/kg intramuscularly or IV 30 minutes before the NAC dose, or droperidol (Inapsine), 1 to 1.5 mg per 20 to 25 lb IV in children aged 2 to 12 years 30 to 60 minutes prior to the NAC dose.

Treatment of hepatic failure is symptomatic and supportive. Early charcoal hemoperfusion initiated prior to stage 4 encephalopathy may increase survival when compared to supportive therapy alone. Consider liver transplantation as a last resort in patients with a poor prognosis due to hepatic failure.

Patient Monitoring: Evaluate the status of the patient's liver function by monitoring aspartate aminotransferase, alanine aminotransferase, bilirubin levels, and prothrombin time. These values should be monitored daily in patients requiring hospitalization. Blood glucose levels should be monitored to detect possible hyperglycemia or hypoglycemia. Monitor urinalysis and renal function test findings. Proteinuria and hematuria may be signs of renal damage. When renal failure is present, the plasma creatinine level rises more rapidly than the level of serum urea nitrogen. A complete blood count and determinations for electrolytes, bicarbonate, and platelets should be obtained. An electrocardiogram and serum amylase concentration should be obtained because of possible myocardial necrosis and pancreatitis.

Enhanced Elimination: Charcoal hemoperfusion, hemodialysis, or forced diuresis are of little value in preventing acetaminophen hepatotoxicity. Hemodialysis may be of benefit as an adjunct in treating hyperammonemia associated with hepatic encephalopathy; it may also be used in treating oliguric renal failure, refractory acidosis, or fluid or electrolyte changes.

References

Peterson RG, Rumack BH. Pharmacokinetics of acetaminophen in children. *Pediatrics.* 1978;62:877-879

Peterson RG, Rumack BH. Toxicity of acetaminophen overdose. *J Am Coll Emerg Phys.* 1978;7:202-205

Rumack BH. Acetaminophen overdose in young children. Treatment and effects of alcohol and other additional ingestants in 417 cases. *AJDC.* 1984;138:428-433

Rumack BH, Matthew H. Acetaminophen poisoning and toxicity. *Pediatrics.* 1975;55:871-876

Rumack BH, Peterson RG. Acetaminophen overdose: incidence, diagnosis, and management in 416 patients. *Pediatrics.* 1978;62:898-903

Rumack BH, Peterson RC, Koch GG, Amara IA. Acetaminophen overdose: 662 cases with evaluation of oral acetylcysteine treatment. *Arch Intern Med.* 1981;141:380-385

Smilkstein MJ, Knapp GL, Kulig KW, Rumack BH. Efficacy of oral *N*-acetylcysteine in the treatment of acetaminophen overdose: analysis of the national multicenter study (1976 to 1985). *N Engl J Med.* 1988;319:1557-1562

Antacids

Available Forms and Sources: The following ingredients may be contained in antacid products: aluminum carbonate, aluminum hydroxide, aluminum phosphate, calcium carbonate, magnesium carbonate, magnesium hydroxide, magnesium oxide, and magnesium trisilicate. They may be formulated as tablets, liquids, gel caps, and chewable dosage forms. Combinations of the above ingredients are common and may also contain simethicone as an anti-gas agent.

Mechanism of Toxicity: These agents can cause mild gastrointestinal irritation when ingested in large quantities.

Toxic Dose: Single large ingestions are easily tolerated and considered nontoxic. Repeated, chronic high doses can produce metabolic alkalosis. Hypernatremia and hypermagnesemia may result from repeated dosing, especially in patients with renal impairment.

Signs and Symptoms: Ingestion of large quantities of these products may cause minor gastrointestinal discomfort including nausea, vomiting, and/or diarrhea.

Diagnostic Testing: These agents are not detected with routine drug screening. No specific testing is necessary.

General Treatment: Dilution with small amounts of clear fluids may provide some relief of gastrointestinal discomfort.

Decontamination: Emesis, gastric lavage, or activated charcoal treatment is not necessary following the ingestion of these agents.

Antidote: No specific antidotes are available.

Specific Treatment: Symptomatic treatment is all that is necessary.

Patient Monitoring: Monitor levels of serum sodium and magnesium following chronic ingestions in patients with renal impairment.

Enhanced Elimination: Enhanced elimination techniques are of no proven value unless electrolyte imbalance cannot be corrected by conventional means.

References

Brand JM, Green FR. Hypermagnesemia and intestinal perforation following antacid administration in a premature infant. *Pediatrics.* 1990; 85:121-124

American Academy of Pediatrics, Committee on Nutrition. Aluminum toxicity in infants and children. *Pediatrics.* 1986;78:1150-1154

Antibiotics - Oral

Available Forms and Sources: Penicillins include amoxicillin, ampicillin, dicloxacillin, and penicillin V; cephalosporins—cefaclor (Ceclor), cefadroxil (Duricef), cefixime (Suprax), cefpodoxime (Vantin), cefprozil (Cefzil), cephalexin (Keflex), cephradine (Velosef), and loracarbef (Lorabid); macrolide antibiotics—azithromycin (Zithromax), clarithromycin (Biaxin), and erythromycin; tetracyclines—doxycycline (Vibramycin), minocycline (Minocin), and tetracycline; sulfonamides—sulfamethoxazole (alone or in combination with trimethoprim), sulfadiazine, and sulfasalazine; and fluoroquinolones—ciprofloxacin (Cipro), enoxacin (Penetrex), lomefloxacin (Maxaquin), norfloxacin (Noroxin), and ofloxacin (Floxin). Penicillins are also available in combination with agents that inactivate β-lactamase enzymes, such as sulbactam and clavulinic acid.

Mechanism of Toxicity: Penicillins and cephalosporins most often produce hypersensitivity reactions. In some cases direct neurotoxicity and nephrotoxicity have been implicated, particularly in the setting of high serum concentrations.

Erythromycin is a gastric irritant and may cause pancreatitis and cholestasis through uncertain mechanisms. Tetracyclines interfere with the deposition of calcium in ossifying bone. Sulfonamides precipitate in the kidneys at high concentrations and also cause hypersensitivity reactions. In addition they produce hemolysis in patients with certain types of glucose-6-phosphate dehydrogenase deficiency. Reversible leukopenia has been reported following trimethoprim-sulfamethoxazole use. Fluoroquinolones cause arthropathy, cartilaginous lesions, and osteochondrosis.

Toxic Dose: Antibiotics intended for oral use generally have a high therapeutic index, making the development of dose-related toxicity unlikely unless massive doses have been ingested. Acute single ingestions are considered nontoxic.

Signs and Symptoms: The most common manifestations following the ingestion of large quantities of oral antibiotics are gastrointestinal, including nausea, vomiting, and diarrhea. These symptoms are usually mild and self-limiting.

Penicillin-class antibiotics may cause hypersensitivity reactions, including urticaria, respiratory distress, and hypotension in susceptible individuals. Interstitial nephritis, with hematuria, oliguria, and possibly an abnormal electrolyte profile, has been reported on a dose-dependent basis following amoxicillin therapy and on a nondose-dependent basis following nafcillin therapy.

Cephalosporins may induce hypersensitivity reactions. Cefaclor has been reported to cause a serum sickness-like illness more commonly than most oral penicillins or other cephalosporins, with skin rashes and arthralgias, in up to 0.5% of recipients.

Cholestatic jaundice has been reported following erythromycin use, particularly after ingestion of erythromycin estolate, but is not expected to result from single acute overdoses. Pancreatitis has been reported.

Sulfonamides may cause hypersensitivity reactions. When serum concentrations of a given sulfonamide exceed its solubility, precipitation may occur within the kidneys, resulting in renal dysfunction. In patients with certain types of glucose-6-phosphate dehydrogenase deficiency, hemolysis may occur following sulfonamide use. Reversible leukopenia has been reported following trimethoprim-sulfamethoxazole use.

Tetracycline causes tooth discoloration in patients whose dentition is not yet fully formed. Discoloration is not a concern following a single exposure. Benign intracranial hypertension has been observed following acute overdose.

One case of acute oliguric renal failure has been reported following a massive exposure to ciprofloxacin.

Diagnostic Testing: These agents are not detected with routine drug screening. Specific measurements of serum drug concentrations are not clinically useful.

General Treatment: Significant symptoms are not anticipated.

Decontamination: (Refer to the treatment section p 6 for the appropriate use of these techniques.) Emesis, gastric lavage, or activated charcoal are generally not necessary unless a massive dose has been ingested.

Antidote: No specific antidotes are available.

Specific Treatment: Rehydrate the patient and correct electrolyte imbalances if vomiting and diarrhea persist. Adequate hydration should be maintained especially following sulfonamide ingestion. Allergic reactions should be treated with standard therapy.

Patient Monitoring: Following large ingestions of penicillin-class agents, microscopic and biochemical urine studies assist in ascertaining the presence or absence of nephritis. After ingestion of tetracyclines or erythromycins, assessment of electrolyte levels and renal and hepatic function is desirable. Following ingestion of sulfonamides, assessment of urine for crystalluria may be appropriate; assessment of leukocyte counts, renal function, and (in susceptible patients) hemoglobin levels may be indicated. After ingestion of fluoroquinolones, renal function may need to be assessed.

Enhanced Elimination: Extracorporeal removal of these agents is usually not necessary following single acute ingestions. It may be necessary following long-term dosing, especially for patients with diminishing renal function. Hemodialysis is effective in removing most penicillins and cephalosporins. Erythromycins and tetracyclines are not removed by hemodialysis. Sulfonamides are generally dialyzable, but dialysis is usually not indicated in the absence of severe renal dysfunction.

References

Geller RJ, Chevalier RL, Spyker DA. Acute amoxicillin nephrotoxicity following an overdose. *Clin Toxicol.* 1986;24:175-182

Hama R, Mori K. High incidence of anaphylactic reactions to cefaclor. *Lancet.* 1988;1:1331

Gumaste VV. Erythromycin induced pancreatitis. *Am J Med.* 1989;86:725

Swanson-Biearman B, Dean BS, Lopez G, Krenzelok EP. The effects of penicillin and cephalosporin ingestions in children less than six years of age. *Vet Hum Toxicol.* 1988;30:66-67

Anticholinergics

Available Forms and Sources: Atropine, scopolamine, and jimson weed produce pure anticholinergic effects. Cyclic antidepressants (see p 46), antihistamines (see p 48), and phenothiazines (see p 50) also produce anticholinergic effects.

Mechanism of Toxicity: The toxicity of anticholinergics results from the blockade of peripheral and central cholinergic receptors.

Toxic Dose: The toxic dose varies and is poorly defined.

Signs and Symptoms: Anticholinergic effects include dry mouth, dry flushed skin, mydriasis, blurred vision, urinary retention, orthostatic hypotension, tachycardia, dysrhythmias, confusion, disorientation, hallucinations, seizures, and coma.

Diagnostic Testing: The naturally occurring agents generally are not detected in a routine drug screen. Monitoring blood levels of these drugs is not clinically useful.

General Treatment: Significant symptoms may occur and life support measures should be instituted as necessary.

Decontamination: (Refer to the treatment section p 6 for the appropriate use of these techniques.) Emesis may be indicated if treatment is initiated within 2 hours of the exposure and the patient is asymptomatic. Activated charcoal may be of value if administered less than 4 hours after ingestion. Because anticholinergic agents decrease bowel activity, activated charcoal should be used with caution in patients with diminished or absent bowel sounds. Repeated doses of activated charcoal are not recommended.

Antidote: Physostigmine is not routinely recommended but may be considered for the occasional uncontrollable and combative patient with predominant anticholinergic signs and symptoms who is at risk for self-injury or injury to others (**see Table 2, p 16, for specific dosing**).

Specific Treatment: Hypotension usually responds to bolus crystalloid therapy, but if this treatment is unsuccessful, administer pressors. Dysrhythmias of uncomplicated anticholinergic toxicity are typically supraventricular and rarely require intervention. Seizures can be treated with benzodiazepines. Respiratory failure is treated with intubation and ventilation.

Patient Monitoring: Monitor the patient's level of consciousness, cardiac rate and rhythm, and blood pressure.

Enhanced Elimination: Enhanced elimination techniques are not of value.

References

Klein-Schwartz W, Oderda GM. Jimson weed intoxication in adolescents and young adults. *AJDC.* 1984;138:737-739

Lauwers LF, Daelemans R, Baute L, Verbraeken H. Scopolamine intoxications. *Intensive Care Med.* 1983;9:283-285

Antidepressants (Excluding MAO Inhibitors)

Available Forms and Sources: The tricyclic antidepressants include amitriptyline (Elavil), nortriptyline (Pamelor), imipramine (Tofranil), doxepin (Sinequan), trimipramine (Surmontil), and desipramine (Norpramin). The tetracyclic antidepressants include amoxapine (Asendin) and maprotiline (Ludiomil). Other unique structures include trazodone (Desyrel), fluoxetine (Prozac), sertraline (Zoloft), paroxetine (Paxil), and bupropion (Wellbutrin). The monoamine oxidase (MAO) inhibitors are discussed in a separate section. Antidepressant compounds are the most frequently involved drugs in serious intoxications because of their inherent toxicity and because they are frequently prescribed.

Mechanism of Toxicity: The toxicity of the tricyclic antidepressant compounds is mediated by their anticholinergic effects, quinidine-like effects on cardiac conduction, direct α-receptor blockade, and inhibition of catecholamine reuptake in the central nervous system and peripheral nervous system. Fluoxetine, sertraline, and paroxetine mainly modify serotonin reuptake.

Toxic Dose: Because of the serious nature of this exposure, the ingestion of even small quantities of these agents requires health care facility evaluation and treatment. The toxic dose is variable, however, for amitriptyline and imipramine—10 to 20 mg/kg may be life-threatening.

Signs and Symptoms: Cyclic antidepressant intoxication may progress rapidly, beginning with anticholinergic signs and progressing to lethal dysrhythmias and hypotension. Early signs and symptoms include drowsiness, dry mucous membranes, mydriasis, hyperreflexia, hypertension, tachycardia, agitation rapidly progressing to coma, seizures, wide QRS complex dysrhythmias, and hypotension.

Amoxapine causes severe epileptogenic effects in the absence of cardiovascular effects. Fluoxetine may produce tachycardia and central nervous system depression but does not tend to produce either seizures or serious cardiovascular effects. The effects of ingestion of sertraline and paroxetine are not well documented.

Diagnostic Testing: Many of these compounds are detected on a routine drug screen. In general, serum concentrations of cyclic antidepressants in excess of 500 ng/mL are associated with toxicity. An electrocardiogram revealing a widened QRS complex together with a consistent history and clinical signs and symptoms may establish the diagnosis of cyclic antidepressant toxicity.

General Treatment: Because significant symptoms are possible, the need for life-support measures, including cardiorespiratory support and seizure control, should be anticipated.

Decontamination: (Refer to the treatment section p 6 for the appropriate use of these techniques.) Because of the rapid onset and progression of symptoms, emesis is not recommended. In patients with altered sensorium, activated charcoal with or without gastric lavage may be used; prior intubation is recommended to avoid aspiration.

Antidote: Physostigmine is not recommended because it is associated with fatal bradydysrhythmias and refractory seizures.

Specific Treatment: Alkalinization of the serum using sodium bicarbonate or hyperventilation appears to exert beneficial effects on cardiac conduction, although data obtained from studies using animals suggest that sodium bicarbonate may be preferable. Prophylactic intravenous bicarbonate is recommended to prevent dysrhythmias. Avoid antidysrhythmics that interfere with conduction, such as quinidine, procainamide, and disopyramide. Hypotension can be treated with fluid volume expansion, followed by inotropic support. The use of dopamine and norepinephrine have both been advocated to reverse the combination of myocardial depression and α-blockade induced hypotension. Extraordinary measures such as use of an intraaortic balloon pump or cardiopulmonary bypass have not been studied, but may be considered in extreme cases.

Patient Monitoring: Monitor cardiac, respiratory, and electrolyte status.

Enhanced Elimination: Enhanced elimination techniques are of no proven value.

References

Borys DJ, Setzer SC, Ling LJ, Reisdorf JJ, Day LC, Krenzelok EP. Acute fluoxetine overdose: a report of 234 cases. *Am J Emerg Med.* 1992;10:115-120

Borys DJ, Setzer SC, Ling LJ, Reisdorf JJ, Day LC, Krenzelok EP. The effects of fluoxetine on the overdose patient. *J Toxicol Clin Toxicol.* 1990;28:331-340

Shannon M, Merola J, Lovejoy FH. Hypotension in severe tricyclic antidepressant overdose. *Am J Emerg Med.* 1988;6:439-442

Vernon DD, Banner W, Garrett JS, Dean JM. Efficacy of dopamine and norepinephrine for treatment of hemodynamic compromise in amitriptyline intoxication. *Crit Care Med.* 1991;19:544-549

Walsh DM. Cyclic antidepressant overdose in children: a proposed treatment protocol. *Pediatr Emerg Care.* 1986;2:28-35

Antihistamines

Available Forms and Sources: Antihistamines are available as single agents or in combination cough and cold preparations. Some are available over-the-counter. Those agents that act centrally and peripherally include diphenhydramine (Benadryl), clemastine (Tavist), tripelennamine (PBZ), pyrilamine (Rynatan), chlorpheniramine (Chlor-Trimeton), brompheniramine (Dimetapp), triprolidine (Actifed), hydroxyzine (Atarax), and promethazine (Phenergan). Those that act primarily peripherally include astemizole (Hismanal), terfenadine (Seldane), and loratadine (Claritin).

Mechanism of Toxicity: The toxicity of antihistamines is primarily due to their anticholinergic actions. Target organs are the brain and the heart. Since astemizole and terfenadine do not penetrate the central nervous system, toxicity is limited to the cardiovascular system.

Toxic Dose: The toxic dose varies from drug to drug. As a general rule, acute ingestion of greater than five times the daily therapeutic dose requires treatment. Young children seem to be very sensitive to relatively smaller doses of astemizole, which can produce life-threatening cardiac dysrhythmias.

Signs and Symptoms: Small to moderate overdoses produce drowsiness, dry mouth, dilated pupils, tachycardia, nausea, and vomiting. Larger overdoses may result in hyperpyrexia, central nervous system depression or stimulation, coma, seizures, hallucinations, and cardiac dysrhythmias. Children are especially sensitive to astemizole and require hospital admission for cardiac monitoring.

Diagnostic Testing: Most of these agents are detected on a routine drug screen. Serum levels are not readily available and do not correlate with toxicity.

General Treatment: Because significant symptoms are possible, the need for life-support measures, including cardiorespiratory support and seizure control, should be anticipated.

Decontamination: (Refer to the treatment section p 6 for the appropriate use of these techniques.) Emesis can be used if instituted early after the exposure and a potentially toxic dose has been ingested. Gastric lavage or activated charcoal treatment is also effective.

Antidote: Physostigmine is not recommended except for the occasional uncontrollable, combative, hallucinating patient at risk for self-injury or injury to others.

Specific Treatment: Seizures can be treated with benzodiazepines. Cardiac dysrhythmias can be treated with an appropriate antidysrhythmic agent or with electrical pacing.

Patient Monitoring: Monitor the patient's level of consciousness and cardiovascular status.

Enhanced Elimination: Enhanced elimination techniques are of no proven value.

References

Hestand HE, Teske DW. Diphenhydramine hydrochloride intoxication. *J Pediatr.* 1977;90:1017-1018

Koppel C, Ibe K, Tenczer J. Clinical symptomatology of diphenhydramine overdose. An evaluation of 136 cases in 1982 to 1985. *Clin Toxicol.* 1987;25:53-70

Magera BE, Betlach CJ, Sweatt AP, Derrick CW Jr. Hydroxyzine intoxication in a 13 month-old child. *Pediatrics.* 1981;67:280-283

Wiley JF, Gelber ML, Henretig FM, Wiley CC, Sandhu S, Loiselle J. Cardiotoxic effects of astemizole overdose in children. *J Pediatr.* 1992;120:799-802

Antipsychotic Agents (Including Phenothiazines and Other Drugs)

Available Forms and Sources: These agents are available as single agents in tablets, capsules, or liquid preparations. Perphenazine is also available in combination with the cyclic antidepressant agent amitriptyline (Triavil).

Phenothiazine-type agents include chlorpromazine (Thorazine), fluphenazine (Prolixin), perphenazine (Trilafon), prochlorperazine (Compazine), trifluoperazine (Stelazine), acetophenazine (Tindal), thioridazine (Mellaril), and mesoridazine (Serentil).

Other nonphenothiazine antipsychotics include haloperidol (Haldol), clozapine (Clozaril), loxapine (Loxitane), molindone (Moban), chlorprothixene (Taractan), and thiothixene (Navane).

Mechanism of Toxicity: The toxicity of the antipsychotics is a result of dopaminergic receptor blockade in the central nervous system, cholinergic receptor blockade in the central nervous system and peripheral nervous system, peripheral α-receptor blockade, and quinidine-like effects. The predominant effect varies among agents. Neuroleptic malignant syndrome has also been reported (see pp 88-89). Clozapine has anticholinergic properties, but little antidopaminergic activity.

Toxic Dose: Toxic doses are not well defined.

Signs and Symptoms: Extrapyramidal signs predominate and include dystonic reactions, torticollis, opisthotonos, akathisia, akinesia, and oculogyric crisis. Dystonic reactions have been seen at therapeutic doses, although overdoses produce the symptom more often. Hyperreflexia, spasticity, and extensor plantar reflexes may occur. The level of consciousness may fluctuate; sedation and coma may occur. Respiratory depression is uncommon and suggests that other drugs have been ingested.

Cardiovascular changes are divided into three groups according to mechanism. Supraventricular tachycardia occurs with many of these compounds secondary to their anticholinergic activity. Orthostatic hypotension occurs, primarily with chlorpromazine and clozapine, due to peripheral α-adrenergic blockade. A quinidine-like disturbance in electrophysiologic function of the myocardium, especially with thioridazine and mesoridazine, leads to prolongation of the QRS and QTc intervals, and ventricular dysrhythmias may occur, including ventricular tachycardia. Atypical ventricular tachycardia (*torsade de pointes*) has been seen in adults.

Pupillary changes occur according to the balance of pharmacologic activity of the particular compound. Chlorpromazine has stronger α-adrenergic blocking properties than anticholinergic activity, so the pupils are small. With the fluphenazine group, pupils are more likely to be large.

Sleep apnea has been reported in infants following therapeutic use.

Diagnostic Testing: Most of these agents are detected on a routine drug screen. Quantitative serum levels are not of value. Some phenothiazines may cross-react with enzyme multiplied immunoassay technique (EMIT) tests for cyclic antidepressants. Phenothiazines are radiopaque, so shadows on the abdominal roentgenogram may support clinical suspicion of the causative agent.

General Treatment: Because significant symptoms are possible, the need for life-support measures, including cardiovascular monitoring, should be anticipated.

Decontamination: (Refer to the treatment section p 6 for the appropriate use of these techniques.) Emesis is not recommended because of the rapid onset of drowsiness and dystonic reactions. Activated charcoal with or without gastric lavage can be used. Whole bowel irrigation may be useful when a substantial number of pills are visualized on the roentgenogram.

Antidote: Dystonic reactions respond to diphenhydramine or benztropine (see Table 2, p 16, for specific dosing). Physostigmine use is not recommended.

Specific Treatment: For neuroleptic malignant syndrome, cooling of the body should begin promptly, and treatment with amantadine, bromocriptine, or dantrolene initiated (see pp 88-89).

Patient Monitoring: Monitor the electrocardiogram, blood pressure, temperature, and level of consciousness.

Enhanced Elimination: Enhanced elimination techniques are of no proven value.

References

Knight ME, Roberts RJ. Phenothiazine and butyrophenone intoxication in children. *Pediatr Clin North Am.* 1986;33:299-309

Gupta JM, Lovejoy FH Jr. Acute phenothiazine toxicity in childhood: a five-year survey. *Pediatrics.* 1967;39:771-774

Kahn A, Hasaerts D, Blum D. Phenothiazine-induced sleep apneas in normal infants. *Pediatrics.* 1985;75:844-847

Barbiturates

Available Forms and Sources: Barbiturates comprise a wide range of products that are used as sedatives, anticonvulsants, and anesthetic agents. The principle difference in the various barbiturates relates to their pharmacokinetics (see Table 8). These agents are available in tablet, capsule, and liquid formulations. They are also available in a few combination products.

Table 8. Barbiturates*

Long Acting	Intermediate Acting	Short Acting	Ultra-short Acting
Mephobarbital (Mebaral)	Amobarbital (Amytal)	Pentobarbital (Nembutal)	Methohexital (Brevital)
Metharbital (Gemonil)	Aprobarbital (Alurate)	Secobarbital (Seconal)	Thiopental (Pentothal)
Phenobarbital (Luminal)	Butabarbital (Butisol)		Thiamylal (Surital)

*Adapted from *Facts and Comparisons: Loose-Leaf Drug Information Service*. St Louis, MO; 1993: 274.

Mechanism of Toxicity: Barbiturates are primarily depressants of the central nervous system and cardiovascular system.

Toxic Dose: The acute toxic dose varies for each barbiturate. In general, the shorter acting agents are believed to be more toxic than the longer acting agents. Doses in the range of 5 to 6 mg/kg for any of these agents represent minimal toxic amounts. Since this dose is in the range commonly used as a loading dose for phenobarbital, it represents a conservative recommendation.

Signs and Symptoms: In general, death occurs as a result of respiratory arrest secondary to central nervous system depression. For patients receiving ventilatory support, death may result from cardiovascular depression. Initial signs and symptoms include central nervous system intoxication with depression of coordination, speech, and cognition. In severe overdose, deep tendon and brain stem reflexes may be depressed, but this usually occurs only well after respiratory depression occurs. Blood pressure is initially affected by a decrease in filling pressure from venodilation followed by myocardial and arteriolar compromise. Other incidental findings can include hypoglycemia, the development of bullous skin lesions (not specific to barbiturates), and hypothermia.

Diagnostic Testing: Most barbiturates are detected in routine drug screens. Phenobarbital can be quantitated by most hospital laboratories. Evidence for the presence of mephobarbital or primidone may be found by analyzing for phenobarbital, a primary metabolite of these drugs.

General Treatment: Since respiratory depression is the most common cause of death, intubation should be undertaken to avoid airway compromise or aspiration of stomach contents.

Decontamination: (Refer to the treatment section p 6 for the appropriate use of these techniques.) Emesis may be induced if instituted early after the exposure. Gastric lavage and/or activated charcoal treatment is preferable to emesis.

Antidote: No specific antidotes are available.

Specific Treatment: Hypotension usually is responsive initially to intravascular volume expansion, but for more significant exposures, pressor support may be required. Central venous pressure monitoring may be extremely important to identify those patients who may need more aggressive support. Primidone may crystallize in the urine, and higher urine flow rates must be maintained when toxicity is associated with this compound.

Patient Monitoring: Sequential phenobarbital levels are useful in assessing the efficacy of treatment in patients with significant symptoms. Patients without previous exposure to barbiturates may experience significant symptoms at therapeutic levels, whereas patients tolerant to the drug may show minimal symptoms with levels considerably above the therapeutic range. Monitor central nervous system and cardiovascular status.

Enhanced Elimination: The pKa of phenobarbital is 7.2, suggesting that alkalinization of the urine may promote the urinary excretion of this compound, although the clinical utility of this therapy has been questioned. Multiple-dose charcoal has been shown to enhance the elimination of phenobarbital and may shorten the duration of coma; it is unlikely, however, to alter the need for supportive care. Hemodialysis and charcoal hemoperfusion have been shown to remove phenobarbital. In general, this has been reserved for serum concentrations in excess of 150 µg/mL.

References

Bertino JS, Reed MD. Barbiturate and nonbarbiturate sedative hypnotic intoxication in children. *Pediatr Clin North Am.* 1986;33:703-722

Sedatives and hypnotics. In: *Facts and Comparisons: Loose-Leaf Drug Information Service.* St. Louis, MO; 1993

Benzodiazepines

Available Forms and Sources: These agents can be divided into groups by their duration of action (see Table 9).

Table 9. Benzodiazepines*

Ultra-short Acting (Half-life <10 h)	Short Acting (Half-life 10-24 h)	Long Acting (Half-life >24 h)
Midazolam (Versed)	Alprazolam (Xanax)	Chlordiazepoxide (Librium)
Temazepam (Restoril)	Estazolam (Prosom)	Clorazepate (Tranxene)
Triazolam (Halcion)	Halazepam (Paxipam)	Clonazepam (Klonopin)
	Oxazepam (Serax)	Diazepam (Valium)
	Lorazepam (Ativan)	Flurazepam (Dalmane)
		Prazepam (Centrax)
		Quazepam (Doral)

*Adapted from Ellenhorn MJ, Barceloux DJ. *Medical Toxicology: Diagnosis and Treatment of Human Poisoning.* New York, NY: Elsevier; 1988:581

Mechanism of Toxicity: Benzodiazepines interact with at least two receptors in the central nervous system to produce their pharmacologic and toxic effects. Many benzodiazepines are addictive with long-term use. Withdrawal symptoms may develop in infants born to mothers using benzodiazepines regularly during pregnancy. Benzodiazepines may be human teratogens. They are excreted in breast milk and may produce symptoms in nursing infants.

Toxic Dose: Doses producing significant toxicity are drug and route dependent. Even after a large ingestion symptoms are usually not life threatening, although deaths have been associated with ingestion of as little as 10 times the therapeutic dose of ultra-short acting agents. Children may be more susceptible to the depressant effects of benzodiazepines. Almost all deaths involving benzodiazepines include another central nervous system depressant agent.

Signs and Symptoms: Mild toxicity presents with lethargy, ataxia, and slurred speech. Very large ingestions, particularly of ultra-short acting agents, may lead to coma, respiratory depression, and death. Tachycardia, hypotension, and hypothermia rarely occur. Severe central nervous system depression or other symptoms should prompt a search for other causes, including ingestion of another drug.

Diagnostic Testing: Benzodiazepines may be detected in urine or serum drug screens. Blood levels are not of clinical value.

General Treatment: Treatment is generally supportive using standard techniques and agents.

Decontamination: (Refer to the treatment section p 6 for the appropriate use of these techniques.) Emesis is contraindicated because of the rapid onset of central nervous system depression. Treatment with activated charcoal or lavage should be considered following recent ingestions.

Antidote: Flumazenil (Romazicon) is a benzodiazepine receptor antagonist **(see Table 2, p 16, for specific dosing).** This agent reverses sedation but may not reverse respiratory depression, thus limiting its effectiveness in the treatment of acute overdoses. It may also precipitate seizures in epileptic patients, patients addicted to benzodiazepines, or in patients coingesting cyclic antidepressants.

Specific Treatment: Treatment is supportive. There is no specific treatment.

Patient Monitoring: Monitor the patient's level of consciousness and respiratory status.

Enhanced Elimination: Enhanced elimination techniques are of no proven value.

References

Ellenhorn MJ, Barceloux DJ. *Medical Toxicology: Diagnosis and Treatment of Human Poisoning.* New York, NY: Elsevier; 1988:581

Greenblatt DJ, Woo E, Allen MD, Orsulak PJ, Shader RI. Rapid recovery from massive diazepam overdose. *JAMA.* 1978;240:1872-1874

Olson KR, Yin L, Osterloh J, Tani A. Coma caused by a trivial triazolam overdose. *Am J Emerg Med.* 1985;3:210-211

β-Adrenergic Blockers

Available Forms and Sources: A number of β-adrenergic blockers are available for both systemic and ophthalmologic use. Those used systemically include acebutolol (Sectral), atenolol (Tenormin), betaxolol (Kerlone), bisoprolol (Zebeta), carteolol (Cartrol), esmolol (Brevibloc), labetalol (Normodyne), metoprolol (Lopressor), nadolol (Corgard), penbutolol (Levatol), pindolol (Visken), propranolol (Inderal), sotalol (Betapace), and timolol (Blocadren). Betaxolol, timolol, and levobunolol are also used as ophthalmologic products.

Mechanism of Toxicity: These drugs block β-adrenergic receptors with varying degrees of β_1 selectivity. β-receptor selectivity is often lost after overdose. Propranolol and some other agents in the class depress myocardial contractility and produce central nervous system depression. Pindolol, carteolol, and acebutolol have partial β-agonist properties and may cause hypertension in overdose.

Toxic Dose: Toxic doses depend on the agent involved. When a recommended daily dose exists, ingestion of greater than twice this dose should be considered potentially toxic.

Signs and Symptoms: The two primary target organs are the heart and the respiratory tract. Sinus bradycardia and hypotension are common and may lead to shock. Heart block and other conduction defects may also occur. Bronchospasm may occur, particularly in patients with preexisting reactive airway disease. Other possible findings include central nervous system depression with seizures and respiratory depression, hypoglycemia, and hyperkalemia.

Diagnostic Testing: β-blockers may be detected in some drug screens. Quantitative serum levels are of no clinical value.

General Treatment: Because significant symptoms are possible, the need for life support measures and cardiac monitoring should be anticipated.

Decontamination: (Refer to the treatment section p 6 for the appropriate use of these techniques.) Emesis is not recommended, particularly following propranolol ingestion because of the risk of central nervous system depression. Gastric lavage and activated charcoal can be used.

Antidote: No specific antidotes are available.

Specific Treatment: Bradycardia and hypotension can be treated with atropine or isoproterenol. Refractory hypotension can be treated with glucagon or a cardiac pacemaker. Bronchospasm can be treated with nebulized bronchodilators. Conduction defects may respond to serum alkalinization with sodium bicarbonate.

Patient Monitoring: Continuous cardiac monitoring is recommended for symptomatic patients or for those with a history of substantial ingestion. Arterial blood gases should be monitored in patients with respiratory symptoms.

Enhanced Elimination: Hemodialysis or hemoperfusion may be helpful following severe poisoning with nadolol or atenolol. It is unlikely to be useful for other agents.

References

Heath A. Beta-adrenoceptor blocker toxicity; clinical features and therapy. *Am J Emerg Med.* 1984;2:518-525

Peterson CD, Leader JS, Sterner S. Glucagon therapy for beta-blocker overdose. *Drug Intel Clin Pharm.* 1984;18:394-398

Weinstein RS. Recognition and management of poisoning with beta-adrenergic blocking agents. *Ann Emerg Med.* 1984;13:1123-1131

Caffeine

Available Forms and Sources: Caffeine is available in regular and extended-release tablets, and as an injectable solution. Caffeine is also an ingredient in many cold preparations, analgesics, and stimulants.

Mechanism of Toxicity: Caffeine causes a number of physiologic changes including release of endogenous catecholamines, increased gastric acid production, and central nervous system and cardiac stimulation.

Toxic Dose: Mild toxicity appears at doses as low as 15 mg/kg. In humans, the oral lethal dose is considered to be 150 to 200 mg/kg (approximately 10 g in adolescents and adults). Clinical toxicity is associated with plasma caffeine concentrations of >30 μg/mL.

Signs and Symptoms: Caffeine produces gastrointestinal effects including nausea, vomiting, abdominal pain, and frank hematemesis. Central nervous system manifestations in children include agitation and hyperactivity. Stimulation of central respiratory centers may lead to respiratory alkalosis. With severe intoxication, seizures may develop. Cardiac disturbances include premature ventricular contractions, supraventricular tachycardia, or life-threatening cardiac dysrhythmias such as ventricular tachycardia or fibrillation. Pulmonary disturbances, particularly pulmonary edema, often occur following severe intoxication. Metabolic disturbances such as hyperglycemia, hypokalemia, and metabolic acidosis may develop.

Diagnostic Testing: Caffeine can be detected in most drug screens. Serum caffeine concentrations can be measured and may be helpful in assessing the severity of exposure. Because caffeine is metabolized to theophylline, a serum theophylline level may be obtained.

General Treatment: Because significant symptoms are possible, the need for life support measures should be anticipated following large exposures.

Decontamination: (Refer to the treatment section p 6 for the appropriate use of these techniques.) Emesis can be used if instituted early. Gastric lavage with activated charcoal or activated charcoal alone may be used.

Antidote: No specific antidotes are available.

Specific Treatment: Seizures can be treated with a benzodiazepine or phenobarbital. Phenytoin may be relatively ineffective as an anticonvulsant. Mild cardiac conduction disturbances (eg, premature ventricular beats) usually do not require intervention. More significant disturbances may require the use of antidysrhythmics or cardioversion. Gastrointestinal effects may be ameliorated by the administration of an H_2 antagonist or antacids. Cimetidine therapy is theoretically contraindicated because it competes with methylxanthines for hepatic metabolism.

Patient Monitoring: Monitor cardiac status, electrolyte levels, blood glucose levels, serum pH, creatine phosphokinase levels, calcium levels, arterial blood gas concentrations, and the electrocardiogram.

Enhanced Elimination: Repeated doses of activated charcoal can enhance the elimination of caffeine. Hemodialysis and hemoperfusion rapidly clear caffeine and are generally indicated when serum caffeine concentrations are >100 µg/mL or life-threatening cardiac dysrhythmias or seizures occur regardless of serum concentration.

References

Dalvi RR. Acute and chronic toxicity of caffeine: a review. *Vet Hum Toxicol.* 1986;28:144-150

Dietrich AM, Mortensen ME. Presentation and management of an acute caffeine overdose. *Pediatr Emerg Care.* 1990;6:296-298

Calcium Channel Blockers

Available Forms and Sources: Calcium channel blockers include verapamil (Calan, Isoptin), nifedipine (Procardia, Adalat), nicardipine (Cardene), felodipine (Plendil), isradipine (DynaCirc), nimodipine (Nimotop), and diltiazem (Cardizem). Some agents are available in sustained-release formulations and in combination with diuretics.

Mechanism of Toxicity: Calcium channel blockers, a structurally diverse group of medications, vary in the site of action, electrophysiologic effect on the heart, and the effect on the vasculature. The mechanism of toxicity is an extension of the therapeutic action of calcium channel blockers to reduce the influx of calcium into the myocardium, the smooth muscle cells of the vasculature, and sinus and atrioventricular nodes by blocking the slow cellular calcium channel. This action results in peripheral, systemic, and coronary vasodilation; impaired cardiac conduction (negative chronotrophy); slowed velocity of cardiac electric impulses (negative dromotrophy); and depression of myocardial contractility (negative inotrophy). The therapeutic effects of the calcium channel blockers vary with their selectivity. In overdose, however, the selectivity may be lost.

Toxic Dose: Any dose greater than the usual maximum daily therapeutic dose should be considered potentially toxic and the patient referred for medical evaluation and monitoring. All exposures in pediatric patients and patients with preexisting heart disease should be evaluated.

Signs and Symptoms: The onset of toxicity is 5 minutes for regular preparations and 4 hours for sustained-release preparations. Sustained-release preparations may delay the onset and peak effects of toxicity for 12 to 24 hours after ingestion, with the possibility of developing concretions and prolonged toxicity.

Hypotension and bradycardia, or tachycardia may develop early after ingestion. Hypotension may be more pronounced following nifedipine ingestion. Conduction disturbances may occur within 30 minutes to 5 hours after ingestion. Atrioventricular dissociation, sinus arrest, and asystole have been documented. Prolongation of the PR interval is a constant finding with toxic serum levels. Other findings on electrocardiogram include inverted P waves, heart block, ST depression, and low-amplitude T waves. Atrioventricular block may be delayed 12 to 16 hours after ingestion. Conduction disturbances worsen in the first 6 hours and may last more than 24 hours after ingestion. Hypoperfusion may lead to lactic acidosis. Anuria has been noted.

Headaches occur due to cerebral vasodilation. Mental status changes, refractory seizures, hemiparesis, central nervous system depression, and coma are due to poor cerebral perfusion. Calcium channel blockers inhibit calcium influx into the β-cells of the islets of the pancreas and suppress calcium-dependent insulin release causing hyperglycemia. Calcium channel blockers may precipitate respiratory insufficiency in patients with Duchenne muscular dystrophy. Other effects include gastric distress and pulmonary edema.

Diagnostic Testing: These agents are not routinely identified in a drug screen. Specific plasma concentrations generally are not available. Prolongation of the PR interval on the electrocardiogram probably indicates toxic serum levels.

General Treatment: Because significant symptoms are possible, the need for life support measures, including cardiorespiratory monitoring, should be anticipated. Patients ingesting sustained-release agents should be observed and monitored for at least 24 hours because heart block has been known to develop 12 to 16 hours after ingestion.

Decontamination: (Refer to the treatment section p 6 for the appropriate use of these techniques.) Emesis is not recommended because of the rapid onset of toxicity and the vagal action produced by vomiting. Gastric lavage should be performed with caution for the same reason. Activated charcoal and a cathartic should be administered. Whole bowel irrigation with polyethylene glycol solution may be of value following the ingestion of sustained-release preparations, but its effectiveness has not been investigated.

Antidote: Calcium may reverse depression of the myocardium but may not reverse nodal depression or peripheral vasodilation; however, the literature fails to document consistent improvement with intravenous calcium and controversy exists regarding which preparation to use. Calcium chloride is more predictable in increasing the concentration of extracellular ionized calcium. Calcium preparations should be administered slowly (0.5 to 2 mL/ min minimum), monitoring for dysrhythmias and hypotension **(see Table 3, p 22, for specific dosing).** Because the effects of calcium usually last only about 15 minutes, a continuous infusion may be necessary.

Glucagon produces a positive inotropic and chronotropic effect; however, it has not been consistently successful **(see Table 2, p 16, for specific dosing).**

Amrinone (Inocor) is an inotropic agent that may reverse the negative inotropic effect of calcium channel blockers. The recommended dose is 0.75 to 2.0 mg/kg (0.15 to 0.4 mL/kg) by intravenous bolus followed by an intravenous drip of 5 to 10 µg/kg/min.

Specific Treatment: (See Table 3, p 22, for specific dosing.) If the patient is symptomatic, a cardiology consultation should be obtained to determine whether hemodynamic monitoring and electrical pacing are needed. Consider the use of an external cutaneous pacemaker early. Bradydysrhythmias and conduction defects often require electrical pacing if the patient is hemodynamically unstable. Atropine can be administered but is rarely effective. Isoproterenol should be used with caution because it may cause peripheral vasodilation. Treat hypotension with standard therapy, although patients seldom respond to these measures in severe poisoning. High doses of vasopressors are usually needed. Norepinephrine or epinephrine may be required in cases where there is no response to calcium infusions, but these drugs may contribute to dysrhythmias. Dopamine and dobutamine have not been proven to be effective but may be tried. Extraordinary measures such as an intra-aortic balloon pump or cardiopulmonary bypass have not been studied but may be considered for severe cases. Patients who experience cardiac arrest usually cannot be effectively resuscitated. Hyperglycemia usually does not require insulin therapy and the administration of excessive exogenous insulin should be avoided.

Patient Monitoring: Monitor levels of blood glucose, calcium, electrolytes, arterial blood gases, creatinine, blood urea nitrogen, and the electrocardiogram. Hemodynamic monitoring is necessary in symptomatic patients.

Enhanced Elimination: Multiple-dose activated charcoal may be useful, especially following the ingestion of sustained-release preparations; however, there are no data on its effectiveness. Extracorporeal measures are not effective. Charcoal hemoperfusion is not recommended. Whole bowel irrigation may enhance the removal of sustained-release preparations.

References

Crump BJ, Holt DW, Vale JA. Lack of response to intravenous calcium in severe verapamil poisoning. *Lancet.* 1982;2:939-940

Epstein ML, Kiel LA, Victoria BE. Cardiac decompensation following verapamil therapy in infants with supraventricular tachycardia. *Pediatrics.* 1985;75:737-740

Goenen M, Col J, Compere A, Bonte J. Treatment of severe verapamil poisoning with combined amrinone-isoproterenol therapy. *Am J Cardiol.* 1986;58:1142-1143

Horowitz BZ, Rhee KJ. Massive verapamil ingestion: a report of two cases and a review of the literature. *Am J Emerg Med.* 1989;7:624-631

Lipman J, Jardine I, Roos C, Dreosti L. Intravenous calcium chloride as an antidote to verapamil-induced hypotension. *Intensive Care Med.* 1982;8:55-57

Passal DB, Crespin FH Jr. Verapamil poisoning in an infant. *Pediatrics.* 1984;73:543-545

Spiller HA, Meyers A, Ziemba T, Riley M. Delayed onset of cardiac arrhythmias from sustained-release verapamil. *Ann Emerg Med.* 1991; 20:201-203

Wells TG, Graham CJ, Moss MM, Kearns GL. Nifedipine poisoning in a child. *Pediatrics.* 1990;86:91-94

Wolf LR, Spadafora MP, Otten EJ. Use of amrinone and glucagon in a case of calcium channel blocker overdose. *Ann Emerg Med.* 1993;22:1225-1228

Zaritsky AL, Horowitz M, Chernow B. Glucagon antagonism of calcium channel-blocker induced myocardial dysfunction. *Crit Care Med.* 1988;16:246-251

Camphor

Available Forms and Sources: Camphor is used in many over-the-counter products designed to relieve the symptoms of upper respiratory tract infections as well as topically for the relief of pain. Products containing camphor at concentrations of 4% (40 mg/mL) or greater include Campho-phenique (10.8%), camphor spirits (10%), Vicks VapoSteam (6.2%), Ben-Gay Vaporizing Rub (5%), and Vicks VapoRub (4.8%). Camphorated oil, containing 20% camphor in cottonseed oil, has been banned from the American market because of its toxicity. There is no established medical indication for the use of camphor.

Mechanism of Toxicity: Camphor is a central nervous system stimulant and depressant.

Toxic Dose: Doses between 10 and 30 mg/kg may result in gastrointestinal irritation, sedation, or both. Severe effects have been noted at doses exceeding 60 mg/kg or a single dose of 1 g.

Signs and Symptoms: Adverse effects are typically noted 5 to 90 minutes following ingestion, but may be delayed up to 6 hours. Seizure activity may develop in the absence of prior symptoms. Nausea, vomiting, gagging, and epigastric burning pain may occur. Irritability and sedation have been observed following doses estimated between 10 and 30 mg/kg. Doses of 60 mg/kg or greater have resulted in syncope, seizures (sometimes recurrent), cyanosis, hypotension, dysrhythmias, and, occasionally, death. Fatalities have been generally attributed to status epilepticus or apnea. Symptoms also have been reported following inhalation and topical exposure. Fetotoxicity has been reported following in utero exposures.

Diagnostic Testing: The odor of camphor may be present on the patient's breath following ingestion. No common laboratory tests are available to quantitate serum camphor concentrations, and camphor generally is not detected by routine drug screens.

General Treatment: Because significant symptoms are possible, the need for life support measures including seizure treatment should be anticipated.

Decontamination: (Refer to the treatment section p 6 for the appropriate use of these techniques.) Emesis should be avoided because of the risk of seizures. Activated charcoal may be of value if administered within 2 hours of exposure and is the preferred treatment. Gastric lavage may be useful if instituted very early.

Antidote: No specific antidotes are available.

Specific Treatment: Seizures can be treated with benzodiazepines or barbiturates. Refractory seizures may require additional anticonvulsants or general anesthesia. Dysrhythmias may be treated with appropriate antidysrhythmic agents.

Patient Monitoring: Serum electrolyte levels and arterial blood gases should be monitored in patients with multiple seizures or respiratory insufficiency.

Enhanced Elimination: Hemodialysis is ineffective. Resin hemoperfusion and lipid hemodialysis have been demonstrated to remove camphor; however, the clinical efficacy of these procedures is controversial.

References

American Academy of Pediatrics, Committee on Drugs. Camphor revisited: focus on toxicity? *Pediatrics*. 1994;94:127-128

Antman E, Jacob G, Volpe B, Finkel S, Savona M. Camphor overdosage: therapeutic considerations. *NY State J Med*. 1978;78:896-897

Geller RJ, Spyker DA, Garrettson LK, Rogol AD. Camphor toxicity: development of a triage strategy. *Vet Hum Toxicol*. 1984;26(suppl 2):8-10

Koppel C, Martens F, Schirop T, Ibe K. Hemoperfusion in acute camphor poisoning. *Intensive Care Med.* 1988;14:431-433

Phelan WJ. Camphor poisoning: over-the-counter dangers. *Pediatrics.* 1976;57:428-431

Siegel E, Wason S. Camphor toxicity. *Pediatr Clin North Am.* 1986;33: 375-379

Carbamazepine

Available Forms and Sources: Carbamazepine (Tegretol) is available as regular tablets, chewable tablets, and as a suspension.

Mechanism of Toxicity: The exact mechanism of toxicity is unknown. The clinical picture is similar to that seen with cyclic antidepressants including central nervous system and respiratory depression, anticholinergic symptoms, and cardiac conduction abnormalities.

Toxic Dose: An initial therapeutic loading dose of carbamazepine is 5 to 10 mg/kg. Toxicity should be considered following ingestion above this range. In the chronic use setting, therapeutic doses may result in toxic serum concentrations.

Signs and Symptoms: Carbamazepine is chemically related to the cyclic antidepressants and phenytoin; however, the effects following overdose are not as serious as those seen with the cyclic antidepressants. Following acute ingestion, the toxicity of carbamazepine focuses around the central nervous system and cardiovascular systems. At low concentrations, cerebellar findings and unusual posturing are most common. At higher serum concentrations coma may occur. Increased seizure activity rarely occurs. The cardiovascular system is affected primarily with cardiac dysrhythmias, which are most commonly bradydysrhythmias, or atrioventricular block, and less commonly by effects on ventricular conduction, such as widening of the QRS complex. Hypotension may occur. Respiratory depression may occur, particularly with larger ingestions. Hyponatremia has also been reported to be caused by an antidiuretic hormone-like effect.

Diagnostic Testing: Carbamazepine serum levels are widely available and the drug is usually detected in routine drug screens. In general, toxicity is observed with serum concentrations in excess of 12 µg/mL. Levels greater than 25 µg/mL are associated with more severe toxicity.

General Treatment: The need for intensive monitoring should be anticipated following substantial ingestions.

Decontamination: (Refer to the treatment section p 6 for the appropriate use of these techniques.) Because of the risk of central nervous system and respiratory depression, emesis should not be used. Gastric lavage with activated charcoal or activated charcoal alone can be used.

Antidote: No specific antidotes are available.

Specific Treatment: The similarity of toxicity to that of the cyclic antidepressants suggests that sodium bicarbonate may be useful in treating dysrhythmias, although no reports have documented such an effect. While case reports have suggested that physostigmine may reverse some of the movement disorders associated with overdose, its use is not recommended, particularly in the presence of bradydysrhythmias. Hypotension should be treated with fluids followed by pressors if needed. Extraordinary measures such as use of an intra-aortic balloon pump or cardiopulmonary bypass have not been studied, but may be considered for extreme poisonings.

Patient Monitoring: Measure arterial blood gases if respiratory depression develops. Monitor cardiac status with serial electrocardiograms if indicated.

Enhanced Elimination: Carbamazepine can be removed by charcoal hemoperfusion as well as repeated doses of activated charcoal. The relative benefits of those approaches are not well explored, and both should probably be reserved for more severe cases. Hemodialysis has not proven to be effective.

References

Durelli L, Massazza U, Cavallo R. Carbamazepine toxicity and poisoning: incidence, clinical features and management. *Med Toxicol Adverse Drug Exp.* 1989;4:95-107

Kalaawi MH, Auger LT, Carroll JE, Angelo-Khattar M. Encephalopathy and brain stem dysfunction in an infant with nonaccidental carbamazepine intoxication. *Clin Pediatr.* 1991;30:385-386

Wason S, Baker RC, Carolan P, Seigel R, Druckenbrod RW. Carbamazepine overdose — the effects of multiple dose activated charcoal. *Clin Toxicol.* 1992;30:39-48

Chloral Hydrate

Available Forms and Sources: Chloral hydrate is a sedative and hypnotic agent available as a capsule, solution, and rectal suppository. The common trade names are Noctec and Aquachloral.

Mechanism of Toxicity: Chloral hydrate toxicity results from central nervous system depression, dysrhythmogenic potential, and local corrosive action. Its cardiotoxicity is similar to that of other polychlorinated molecules, eg, trichloroethylene and trichloromethane. Chloral hydrate also causes significant local gastrointestinal irritation.

Toxic Dose: Chloral hydrate can be administered safely over a wide range of doses. The minimal sedating dose in children is 8 to 15 mg/kg. Typical sedating doses are 20 to 25 mg/kg. The hypnotic dose is 25 to 50 mg/kg (although doses as high as 100 mg/kg have been administered without significant adverse effect). Doses greater than 75 mg/kg may be associated with the development of profound central nervous system depression and cardiac dysrhythmias. Death has been reported with chloral hydrate doses as low as 125 mg/kg.

Signs and Symptoms: Central nervous system manifestations predominate, with an obtunded appearance, decreased respiratory effort, miosis, coma, and apnea. Cardiac disturbances include hypotension and conduction abnormalities (ventricular or supraventricular tachydysrhythmias as well as bradydysrhythmias) and may be difficult to treat. A local corrosive effect may lead to erosive gastritis with nausea, vomiting, abdominal pain, and heme-positive emesis or stools. Local necrosis with gastrointestinal perforation has been reported. Hepatic and renal injury may also occur.

Diagnostic Testing: Neither chloral hydrate or its metabolites are detected in a routine drug screen. Chloral hydrate is almost immediately transformed to the active metabolite trichloroethanol, which can be measured in serum and may be monitored in the evaluation of chloral hydrate overdose. Because chloral hydrate is radiopaque, an abdominal radiograph may assist in the evaluation of the ingestion of capsules.

General Treatment: Because significant symptoms are possible, the need for life support measures including respiratory support should be anticipated following substantial ingestions.

Decontamination: (Refer to the treatment section p 6 for the appropriate use of these techniques.) Gastrointestinal decontamination should be instituted in cases of oral overdose; there is no role for decontamination after overdoses by rectal administration. Emesis is not recommended because of the risk of central nervous system depression. Gastric lavage with activated charcoal or activated charcoal alone should be considered if a potentially toxic dose has been ingested.

Antidote: No specific antidotes are available.

Specific Treatment: Cardiac dysrhythmias can be treated using standard antidysrhythmic agents. Hypotension is best treated with fluids; pressors should be used judiciously. Epinephrine treatment theoretically should be avoided because chlorinated compounds such as chloral hydrate increase myocardial sensitivity to catecholamines, potentially precipitating ventricular fibrillation.

Patient Monitoring: Monitor arterial blood gases, serum electrolytes, and the electrocardiogram.

Enhanced Elimination: Hemodialysis and hemoperfusion have been reported to increase the clearance of chloral hydrate and its metabolites. Exchange transfusion is not effective.

References

Graham SR, Day RO, Lee R, Fulde GWO. Overdose with chloral hydrate: a pharmacological and therapeutic review. *Med J Aust.* 1988;149:686-688

Hirsch IA, Zauder HL. Chloral hydrate: a potential cause of arrhythmias. *Anesth Analg.* 1986;65:691-692

Houpt M. Death following oral sedation. *J Dent Child.* 1988;55:123-124

Vaziri ND, Kumar KP, Mirahmadi K, Rosen SM. Hemodialysis in treatment of acute chloral hydrate poisoning. *South Med J.* 1977;70:377-378

Clonidine and Related Centrally Acting Antihypertensives

Available Forms and Sources: Clonidine (Catapres) is available in tablets and as a transdermal "patch." After 11 days of use, patches may still contain as much as 40% of the drug. It is also available in combination with some diuretics. Guanabenz (Wytensin) and guanfacine (Tenex) are available as tablets.

Mechanism of Toxicity: These agents produce central nervous system α_2 agonist effects that result in a reduction of sympathetic outflow from central cardiorespiratory centers, producing a fall in heart rate and blood pressure. They also appear to have agonist action at central nervous system opiate receptors. High doses of clonidine also stimulate peripheral adrenergic receptors, leading to significant increases in blood pressure.

Toxic Dose: Toxicity has been reported after the ingestion of as little as 0.1 to 0.2 mg of clonidine. Severe toxicity has been reported after the ingestion of discarded used clonidine patches. The toxic doses of guanabenz and guanfacine are poorly defined.

Signs and Symptoms: Symptoms may appear within 30 to 60 minutes after ingestion. Central nervous system signs of toxicity are most common with drowsiness, lethargy, stupor, or coma, which may be accompanied by respiratory depression and miosis. Up to 50% of patients with severe intoxication also experience hypothermia.

Cardiovascular signs involve blood pressure instability, which may include initial transient hypertension followed by alternating periods of hypotension and hypertension, depending on the predominance of peripheral as opposed to central nervous system effects. Bradycardia typically accompanies hypotension.

Diagnostic Testing: Clonidine is not usually identified in drug screens. Serum measurements of these agents are not clinically useful.

General Treatment: Because significant symptoms are possible, the need for life support measures including respiratory support should be anticipated. All children ingesting these agents should be referred to a health care facility for evaluation.

Decontamination: (Refer to the treatment section p 6 for the appropriate use of these techniques.) Emesis is contraindicated because of the risk of rapid central nervous system depression. Activated charcoal treatment with or without prior gastric lavage can be considered if instituted early.

Antidote: Naloxone may reverse central nervous system depression; results, however, are inconsistent (see Table 2, p 16, for specific dosing). Large doses (4 to 5 mg in children; 5 to 10 mg in adolescents) may be required. Naloxone should not be used in place of aggressive supportive care.

Specific Treatment: Bradycardia can be treated with atropine and isoproterenol as needed. Hypotension can be treated with standard therapy. Hypertension is transient and rarely requires treatment.

Patient Monitoring: Electrocardiography should be performed to identify the presence of any conduction disturbances. Arterial or capillary blood gases should be monitored if respiratory symptoms occur.

Enhanced Elimination: Enhanced elimination techniques are of no proven value.

References

Artman M, Boerth RC. Clonidine poisoning - a complex problem. *AJDC.* 1983;137:171-174

Bamshad MJ, Wasserman GS. Pediatric clonidine intoxications. *Vet Hum Toxicol.* 1990;32:220-222

Caravati EM, Bennett DL. Clonidine transdermal patch poisoning. *Ann Emerg Med.* 1988;17:175-176

Fiser DH, Moss MM, Walker W. Critical care for clonidine poisoning in toddlers. *Crit Care Med.* 1990;18:1124-1128

Heidemann SM, Sarnaik AP. Clonidine poisoning in children. *Crit Care Med.* 1990;18:618-620

Jensen P, Edgren B, Hall L, Ring JC. Hemodynamic effects following ingestion of an imidazoline-containing product. *Pediatr Emerg Care.* 1989;5:110-112

Wiley JF, Wiley CC, Torrey SB, Henretig FM. Clonidine poisoning in young children. *J Pediatr.* 1990;116:654-658

Contraceptives - Oral

Available Forms and Sources: These products contain either a single progestational agent or more commonly are a combination of an estrogen and progesterone. Some products contain placebos that may have small amounts of iron. The risk of iron toxicity is unlikely from these products.

Mechanism of Toxicity: These agents can produce mild local irritation of the gastric mucosa.

Toxic Dose: There is a wide margin of safety following acute ingestion of these products. A toxic dose has not been established. The ingestion of a 1-month supply (21 to 28 tablets) of an oral contraceptive should cause only minor symptoms.

Signs and Symptoms: Nausea and vomiting are the most common effects observed even following a large ingestion. Minor vaginal bleeding because of hormone withdrawal has been reported in young girls following the ingestion of several tablets.

Diagnostic Testing: These agents are not detected by a routine drug screen. No diagnostic testing is necessary.

General Treatment: Significant acute symptoms are not anticipated. The administration of small amounts of food, fluids, or both can be given to decrease the gastrointestinal effects. Inform the parent about the possibility of minor vaginal bleeding, if appropriate.

Decontamination: Gastrointestinal decontamination is not necessary.

Antidote: No specific antidotes are available.

Specific Treatment: Treatment is supportive. There is no specific treatment.

Patient Monitoring: No specific monitoring is necessary.

Enhanced Elimination: Enhanced elimination techniques are not necessary.

Reference

Picchioni AL. Acute overdose of oral contraceptives. *Am J Hosp Pharm.* 1965;22:486

Cyclobenzaprine

Available Forms and Sources: Cyclobenzaprine (Flexeril) is a skeletal muscle relaxant available as a tablet.

Mechanism of Toxicity: Cyclobenzaprine has anticholinergic, antihistaminic, and sedative properties. It is chemically related to amitriptyline (a cyclic antidepressant); serious cardiac dysrhythmias and seizures, however, have not been reported following overdose.

Toxic Dose: A toxic dose has not been established, and limited data are available. Because children may be more sensitive to the drug than adults, consider observation or evaluation if more than 2 tablets are ingested.

Signs and Symptoms: The onset of symptoms may be delayed up to 8 hours and persist up to 24 hours. Anticholinergic symptoms include dry mouth, tachycardia, flushed skin, decreased gastrointestinal motility, urinary retention, confusion, hallucinations, and sedation.

Diagnostic Testing: Cyclobenzaprine may be identified in routine drug screens. Plasma drug levels are not of value.

General Treatment: Significant acute symptoms are not anticipated.

Decontamination: (Refer to the treatment section p 6 for the appropriate use of these techniques.) Emesis may be of value early after exposure but should be used with caution because of the possibility of drowsiness and the risk of aspiration. If the patient is drowsy, treatment with activated charcoal may be preferred. It should be used with caution if bowel sounds are diminished or absent.

Antidote: Physostigmine can be used to treat symptoms of severe exposures only. Use with caution (see **Table 2, p 16, for specific dosing**).

Specific Treatment: Treatment is supportive. There is no specific treatment.

Patient Monitoring: Monitor mental and cardiac status.

Enhanced Elimination: Repeated doses of activated charcoal may be of value but diminished bowel motility may preclude its use. Hemodialysis or hemoperfusion is of no value.

Reference

O'Riordan W, Gillette P, Calderon J, Stennes RL. Overdose of cyclobenzaprine, the tricyclic muscle relaxant. *Ann Emerg Med.* 1986;15:592-593

Dextromethorphan

Available Forms and Sources: Dextromethorphan is marketed as an antitussive in over-the-counter and prescription products in the United States. Formulations include capsules, tablets, lozenges, and liquids. Sustained-release preparations are available that may contain larger doses. Many products containing dextromethorphan also contain alcohol, which produces an additive central nervous system depressant effect.

Mechanism of Toxicity: Dextromethorphan is an analogue of codeine. It acts on the central nervous system to elevate the cough threshold. Unlike codeine, it has no analgesic properties and is not physiologically addictive.

Toxic Dose: Acute ingestions of more than 10 mg/kg may produce central nervous system depression. Doses as high as 100 times the usual therapeutic dose have not been associated with fatalities.

Signs and Symptoms: Symptoms relate to the central nervous system and include lethargy, dizziness, ataxia, nystagmus, hallucinations, and blurred vision. In severe cases coma and shallow respirations develop. Other symptoms seen occasionally include nausea and vomiting, urticaria, seizures, tachycardia, and hypertension. Long-acting products are likely to produce more marked and prolonged symptoms in children.

Diagnostic Testing: Dextromethorphan and its metabolites are usually detected in blood and urine drug screens. Blood levels are not clinically useful. Because many products containing dextromethorphan also contain acetaminophen and ethanol, consideration should be given to obtaining blood levels of these potential toxins as well.

General Treatment: Significant symptoms are possible, and the need for life support measures including respiratory support should be anticipated following substantial ingestion.

Decontamination: (Refer to the treatment section p 6 for the appropriate use of these techniques.) Emesis should be avoided because of the risk of central nervous system depression. Activated charcoal treatment can be considered if instituted early.

Antidote: Naloxone can reverse central nervous system depression in most cases. Repeated doses or continuous infusion may be required in large ingestions. Patients receiving naloxone should be observed for at least 4 to 6 hours after the last dose for the possible return of symptoms (**see Table 2, p 16, for specific dosing**).

Specific Treatment: Treatment is supportive. There is no specific treatment.

Patient Monitoring: Monitor mental status and respiratory status.

Enhanced Elimination: Enhanced elimination techniques are of no proven value.

References

American Academy of Pediatrics, Committee on Drugs. Use of codeine and dextromethorphan-containing cough syrups in pediatrics. *Pediatrics.* 1978;62:118-122

Shaul WL, Wandell M, Robertson WO. Dextromethorphan toxicity: reversal by naloxone. *Pediatrics.* 1977;59:117-118

Pender ES, Parks BR. Toxicity with dextromethorphan-containing preparations: a literature review and report of two additional cases. *Pediatr Emerg Care.* 1991;7:163-165

Schneider SM, Michelson EA, Boucek CD, Ilkhanipour K. Dextromethorphan poisoning reversed by naloxone. *Am J Emerg Med.* 1991;9:237-238

Digitalis and Other Cardiac Glycosides

Available Forms and Sources: Pharmaceutical preparations include digoxin and digitoxin available as tablets, capsules, and a liquid.

Other cardiac glycosides are found in plants such as digitalis lantana, dogbane (*Apocynum cannabinum*), European mistletoe (*Viscum album*), foxglove (*Digitalis purpurea*), hispidius seeds, lily of the valley (*Convallaria majalis*), oleander (*Nerium oleander*), rhododendron, squill (*Urginea maritima*), wall flower (*Cheiranthus cheiri*), yellow oleander (*Thevetia peruviana*), and in *Bufo* species of toad skin.

Mechanism of Toxicity: Cardiac glycosides inhibit the sodium/potassium-adenosine triphosphate (ATP) pump in cells, leading to intracellular potassium loss. They stimulate phase 4 depolarization, which causes increased automaticity and ectopy. Pacemaker cells are inhibited, and the refractory period is prolonged, leading to various degrees of heart block; vagal tone is increased causing bradycardia.

Toxic Dose: A single ingestion of less than 2 mg in a child rarely causes a serious toxic reaction. A single ingestion of more than 4 mg in children and over 10 mg in adults or adolescents can result in serious toxicity. In patients taking a digitalis product chronically, the acute ingestion of two to three times the therapeutic daily maintenance dose can lead to toxicity. Patients at greater risk for intoxication include those with diminished renal (digoxin) or liver (digitoxin) function, electrolyte disturbances, advanced heart disease or pulmonary disease, or acute myocardial infarction.

Signs and Symptoms: Acute poisoning is more likely to produce bradycardia, various degrees of heart block, and hyperkalemia than chronic toxicity. Infants and children with healthy hearts tolerate overdoses of digoxin remarkably well. Gastrointestinal symptoms, including abdominal pain, nausea, vomiting, and diarrhea, may begin 1 hour after ingestion.

No specific dysrhythmia is characteristic of digitalis toxicity. Changes on the electrocardiogram show ST segment scooping, flattened and inverted T waves, a shortened QT interval, and a prolonged PR interval. Bradydysrhythmias usually occur in patients with healthy hearts and tachydysrhythmias occur in patients with preexisting heart disease. Ventricular tachycardia is only seen with severe poisonings. Life-threatening cardiac symptoms may be delayed for up to 18 hours. In acute ingestion the poor prognostic factors are a serum digoxin level over 15 ng/mL 6 to 8 hours after ingestion and initial hyperkalemia. Hyperkalemia (>5.5 mEq/L) is associated with up to 50% mortality without antibody treatment.

Chronic digitalis intoxication is more likely to produce central nervous system effects such as depression, headache, fatigue, scotoma, blurred vision, color perception disturbances such as yellow vision, halos around lights, delirium, hallucinations, or psychosis. Tachycardia, serious premature ventricular contractions, ventricular dysrhythmias, and hypokalemia are also common.

Diagnostic Testing: Digitalis glycosides are not detected on routine drug screens and specific levels must be measured. Serum digoxin concentrations obtained less than 6 hours after ingestion may not reflect tissue concentrations and may not predict toxicity. A toxic concentration of digoxin is greater than 2.5 ng/mL in adults and over 4 ng/mL in infants; serious toxicity is over 10 ng/mL in adults and over 5 ng/mL in children. Digitoxin is toxic in concentrations over 35 ng/mL. An endogenous digoxin-like immunoreactive substance that cross-reacts with most common immunoassays (but not high-pressure liquid chromatographic assays) may be found in concentrations as high as 4.1 ng/mL in certain patients not exposed to cardiac glycosides. It has been reported in premature and full-term newborns, in patients with chronic renal failure and renal hypertension or abnormal immunoglobin levels, and in women in the third trimester of pregnancy.

The measured serum total protein-bound digoxin increases after administration of digitalis-specific antibodies (Digibind), but the free, active digoxin concentration decreases. Results of standard assays that measure only protein-bound digoxin are abnormal for more than 96 hours after the administration of digitalis-specific antibodies. Digitalis administered after antibody therapy may be bound and inactivated for as long as 1 week (usually 5 to 7 days).

General Treatment: Because significant symptoms are possible, the need for life support measures including cardiac monitoring should be anticipated.

Decontamination: (Refer to the treatment section p 6 for the appropriate use of these techniques.) Emesis should be avoided because vomiting has a vagal effect. Gastric lavage should also be avoided because of its vagal effect. The preferred method of gastrointestinal decontamination is the administration of activated charcoal. If a nasogastric tube is used for charcoal administration, pretreatment with atropine has been suggested to avoid the vagal effect.

Antidote: Digitalis-specific antibodies (Fab fragments of digoxin-specific sheep antibodies [Digibind]) bind digoxin, making it unavailable at sites of action. Consider the administration of Fab fragments for the following: (1) imminent cardiac arrest, shock, or rapid progression of clinical findings—progressive obtundation, worsening conduction defects, rapidly rising serum potassium concentrations ; (2) hyperkalemia (a potassium level >5.5 mEq/L; (3) serum digoxin levels over 10 ng/mL in adults and 5 ng/mL in children at steady state (6 to 8 hours after ingestion). This level indicates the patient is at high risk of developing life-threatening dysrhythmias. Administration should be based on the symptoms, not solely on the serum digoxin level; (4) hemodynamically unstable life-threatening dysrhythmias; (5) ingestion of over 10 mg in adults or over 0.2 mg/kg (4 mg) in children; or (6) bradycardia or second- or third-degree heart block unresponsive to atropine therapy. Fab fragments have also been useful in the treatment of digitoxin intoxication and oleander poisoning (see product literature for specific dosing).

The dose of Fab fragments is based on the amount of digoxin ingested. If the amount ingested is unknown, the dose is based on the clinical condition or the steady-state serum concentration at 6 to 8 hours after ingestion. The product literature gives specific dosing recommendations. Adverse effects are rare and include hypersensitivity reactions, hypokalemia, and worsening of preexisting congestive heart failure. Avoid using Fab fragments and emergency potassium-lowering drugs (bicarbonate or glucose and insulin) concomitantly because severe hypokalemia may develop.

Specific Treatment: (See Tables 2 and 3, pp 16 and 22, respectively, for specific dosing.) Do not administer potassium until the serum potassium level and electrocardiogram have been evaluated. If abnormal cardiac rhythm with instability, peaked T waves, or elevated potassium levels occurs, arrangements should be made to have digoxin-specific Fab fragments and an external cutaneous pacemaker readily available. Avoid class I antidysrhythmic agents (quinidine, procainamide, disopyramide), bretylium, isoproterenol, carotid sinus massage, calcium, β-blockers, and calcium channel blockers.

Treat ventricular dysrhythmias with an appropriate agent such as phenytoin and lidocaine. Magnesium sulfate ($MgSO_4$) is useful in treating idionodal and ventricular tachycardia and atypical ventricular tachycardia, or *torsade de pointes*. The initial dose of $MgSO_4$ in children is 25 to 50 mg/kg and is then titrated to control the dysrhythmia. If there is no evidence of renal failure, administer $MgSO_4$ and monitor the patient with an electrocardiogram and magnesium blood levels. Stop $MgSO_4$ treatment if hypotension, heart block, or decreased deep tendon reflexes develop. Magnesium may stabilize the cardiac status while the patient awaits Fab treatment. *Torsade de pointes* has also been treated effectively with isoproterenol, lidocaine, phenytoin, and atrial or ventricular overdrive pacing to shorten the QT interval. Cardioversion in digitalis intoxication is risky because it tends to produce ventricular fibrillation and should be considered only as a last resort for life-threatening dysrhythmias after phenytoin has been given. Cardioversion should be administered at reduced power settings starting at 5 to 10 J. The need for higher power settings indicates the need for lidocaine before further attempts at cardioversion are made.

Treat hemodynamically unstable bradycardia and heart block with either atropine or low-dose phenytoin. If the response to atropine or phenytoin is inadequate or high-grade block is present, an external cutaneous temporary pacemaker should be seriously considered, although serious intoxications may not respond to pacemakers. Do not treat with isoproterenol because it may cause dysrhythmias.

Initial treatment of hyperkalemia can include glucose and insulin infusions and sodium polystyrene sulfonate (Kayexalate). These interventions should not be administered with Fab fragments because severe, life-threatening hypokalemia may result.

Patient Monitoring: Monitor the electrocardiogram. Determine levels of electrolytes, blood glucose, magnesium, serum urea nitrogen, creatinine, and calcium and correct any abnormalities as necessary. Low magnesium and potassium levels and high calcium and sodium levels increase digitalis toxicity. Serial electrolyte and renal function monitoring is advised for at least 24 to 48 hours after ingestion. Monitor patients with significant ingestions 18 to 24 hours for dysrhythmias because digitalis preparations have long half-lives.

Enhanced Elimination: Repeated doses of activated charcoal are recommended because they may interrupt enterohepatic recirculation. Enhanced elimination techniques are of no proven value to remove digitalis glycosides but may be of value to correct hyperkalemia.

References

Antman EM, Wenger TL, Butler VP Jr, Haber E, Smith TW. Treatment of 150 cases of life-threatening digitalis intoxication with digoxin-specific Fab antibody fragments: final report of a multicenter study. *Circulation.* 1990;81:1744-1752

Boldy DA, Smart V, Vale JA. Multiple doses of charcoal in digoxin poisoning. *Lancet.* 1985;2:1076-1077

Green SM, Naftel J. Antiarrhythmic efficacy of magnesium in the setting of life-threatening digoxin toxicity. *Am J Emerg Med.* 1989;7:347-348

Kaufman J, Leikin J, Kendzierski D, Polin K. Use of digoxin FAB immune fragments in a seven-day-old infant. *Pediatr Emerg Care.* 1990;6:118-121

Lewander WJ, Gaudreault P, Einhorn A, Henretig FM, Lacouture PG, Lovejoy FH Jr. Acute pediatric digoxin ingestion. *AJDC.* 1986; 140:770-773

Smith TW, Butler VP Jr, Haber E, et al. Treatment of life-threatening digitalis intoxication with digoxin-specific Fab antibody fragments: experience in 26 cases. *N Engl J Med.* 1982;307:1357-1362

Stone J, Bentur Y, Zalstein E, et al. Effect of endogenous digoxin-like substances on the interpretation of high concentrations of digoxin in children. *J Pediatr.* 1990;117:321-325

Tzivioni D, Banai S, Schuger C, et al. Treatment of torsade de pointes with magnesium sulfate. *Circulation.* 1988;77:392-397

Woolf AD, Wenger T, Smith TW, et al. The use of digoxin-specific FAB fragments for severe digitalis intoxication in children. *N Engl J Med.* 1992;326:1739-1744

Woolf A. Revising the management of digitalis poisoning. *J Toxicol Clin Toxicol.* 1993;31:275-276

Diuretics

Available Forms and Sources: Thiazide diuretics include chlorothiazide (Diuril), hydrochlorothiazide (Esidrix, Hydro-DIURIL), chlorthalidone (Hygroton), metolazone (Zaroxolyn), and indapamide (Lozol). Loop diuretics include furosemide (Lasix) and bumetanide (Bumex). Potassium-sparing diuretics include triamterene (Dyrenium and many combination products), amiloride (Midamor) and spironolactone (Aldactone). These agents are formulated in tablets, capsules, and liquids as single agents or in combination with a variety of antihypertensive agents.

Mechanism of Toxicity: The toxic effects are an extension of the pharmacologic effects of these agents. The degree of fluid and electrolyte loss depends on the site of action of the individual agent in the nephron.

Toxic Dose: Toxic doses are not well defined in the literature. Generally, five times the maximum daily dose of an agent may require intervention.

Signs and Symptoms: Nausea, vomiting, weakness, and drowsiness have been reported following the ingestion of thiazide diuretics. Early reports describe lethargy and coma in two children following the ingestion of 15 g of chlorthalidone without evidence of significant fluid and electrolyte loss. Thiazides can produce significant hyperglycemia. Hypokalemia and hyponatremia may occur. Fluid and electrolyte imbalance can occur but is unlikely following acute ingestions.

Diagnostic Testing: These agents are not routinely identified in a drug screen.

General Treatment: Significant acute symptoms are not anticipated.

Decontamination: (Refer to the treatment section p 6 for the appropriate use of these techniques.) Gastrointestinal decontamination is not necessary unless very large quantities of an agent have been ingested. Emesis can be used if instituted early. Gastric lavage and/or activated charcoal may also be used.

Antidote: No specific antidotes are available.

Specific Treatment: Replace fluid and electrolytes (sodium and potassium) as necessary.

Patient Monitoring: Monitor electrolytes and fluid balance if significant diuresis occurs.

Enhanced Elimination: Enhanced elimination techniques are of no proven value.

Reference

Bass JW, Beisel WR. Coma due to acute chlorothiazide intoxication. *AJDC.* 1963;106:620-623

Fluoride

Available Forms and Sources: Fluoride is a dental care supplement most commonly found in the form of sodium fluoride. One gram of sodium fluoride yields 452 mg of fluoride ion. Oral products include sodium fluoride solutions, tablets, and vitamins with fluoride as tablets or drops. Topical products include toothpastes, gels, and rinses.

Fluoride is also found in insecticides (which may contain 65% to 95% sodium fluoride), preservatives (which may contain 60% to 95% sodium or calcium fluoride), and drinking water. Water fluoridation is the process of adjusting the fluoride content of fluoride-deficient water to the recommended level for optimal dental health. Ideally, the fluoride content of the local water supply should be adjusted to a level between 0.7 and 1.0 parts per million (1 ppm = 1 mg/L). Ingestion of water containing fluoride at these levels does not produce acute or chronic toxicity.

Mechanism of Toxicity: After acute overdose, fluoride produces a number of toxic actions, the most important of which is its ability to bind calcium, resulting in hypocalcemia, enzyme inhibition, cardiac conduction disturbances, coagulopathy, and cell death. With its potent affinity for calcium ion, fluoride disturbs all metabolic actions requiring calcium as a cofactor. As an inhibitor of glycolytic enzymes, it can impair glucose homeostasis. In the gastrointestinal tract, fluoride ion in association with hydrogen ion creates hydrogen fluoride, a potent acid that can result in significant gastrointestinal epithelial injury.

Toxic Dose: Ingestions of 3 to 5 mg/kg of fluoride ion are associated with nausea, vomiting, and fatigue in 30% to 35% of children. Ingestions of 5 to 10 mg/kg invariably cause symptoms. Death generally occurs with ingestions of 30 to 60 mg/kg, although doses as low as 16 mg/kg have been associated with fatalities.

Signs and Symptoms: Acute fluoride intoxication manifests with gastrointestinal, metabolic, cardiac, musculoskeletal, hematologic, and neurologic symptoms. These effects typically begin to appear within 1 hour of ingestion.

Gastrointestinal effects include local irritation with nausea, vomiting, abdominal cramps, and hematemesis. Fluoride induces a number of electrolyte disturbances including hypocalcemia, hypomagnesemia, and hyperkalemia. Cardiac effects consist of conduction disturbances that cause tachydysrhythmias and vasomotor instability. Conduction changes include a prolonged QT interval secondary to hypocalcemia. Peaked T waves associated with hyperkalemia may also appear. Fluoride intoxication may cause hypotension through vascular smooth muscle relaxation as well as direct myocardial depression. Musculoskeletal disturbances occur secondary to hypocalcemia and include tetany, muscle weakness, and respiratory paralysis. Coagulation disturbances can also occur with hypocalcemia, resulting in bleeding diatheses. Manifestations of toxicity may continue as long as 24 hours after ingestion. Central nervous system changes are rare and typically result from inadequate cerebral perfusion or glucose disturbances. Seizures may occur.

Long-term exposure to excessive fluoride (fluorosis) may be associated with dental and skeletal disturbances.

Diagnostic Testing: Fluoride is not detected on a routine drug screen. Normal serum fluoride concentrations are 0.04 to 0.2 µg/mL and acute toxicity is associated with serum fluoride levels of >2 μg/mL. Levels are not usually available emergently and are of limited clinical value.

General Treatment: Because significant symptoms are possible, the need for life support measures including respiratory support and cardiac monitoring should be anticipated following very large ingestions.

Decontamination: (Refer to the treatment section p 6 for the appropriate use of these techniques.) Emesis can be used if instituted early and gastric lavage may be considered if a potentially toxic dose has been ingested. Activated charcoal does not effectively bind fluoride.

Antidote: Following ingestions of >10 mg/kg, a bolus dose of calcium should be given empirically. If clinical evidence of hypocalcemia is present, the bolus should be followed by a continuous infusion of 10% calcium gluconate at a dose of 150 mL/M^2/d (see Table 3, p 22, for specific dosing).

Specific Treatment: (See Table 3, p 22, for specific dosing.) Hypotension may require fluids and vasopressors. Sodium polystyrene sulfonate (Kayexalate) or hemodialysis may be needed to treat severe hyperkalemia. All patients with symptomatic hypocalcemia require cardiac monitoring. Treatment of cardiac dysrhythmias may require intravenous lidocaine, cardioversion, or both.

Patient Monitoring: Serum electrolytes, calcium, and magnesium levels should be closely monitored. An electrocardiogram should be monitored in symptomatic patients.

Enhanced Elimination: Because fluoride is excreted renally, a fluid diuresis should be initiated to maintain urine output at >2 mL/kg/h. Hemodialysis may remove as much as 30% of a fluoride burden in addition to correcting electrolyte disturbances; its use, however, is rarely necessary.

References

American Academy of Pediatrics, Committee on Nutrition. Fluoride supplementation. *Pediatrics*. 1986;77:758-761. Under revision

Augenstein WL, Spoerke DG, Kulig KW, et al. Fluoride ingestion in children: a review of 87 cases. *Pediatrics*. 1991;88:907-912

Cummings CC, McIvor ME. Fluoride-induced hyperkalemia: the role of Ca^{2+} dependent K^+ channels. *Am J Emerg Med*. 1988;6:1-3

Ekstrand J. Pharmacokinetic aspects of topical fluorides. *J Dent Res*. 1987;66:1061-1065

McIvor ME, Cummings CE, Mower MM, et al. Sudden cardiac death from acute fluoride intoxication: the role of potassium. *Ann Emerg Med*. 1987;16:777-781

Monsour PA, Kruger BJ, Petrie AF, McNee JL. Acute fluoride poisoning after ingestion of sodium fluoride tablets. *Med J Aust*. 1984;141:503-505

Haloperidol

Available Forms and Sources: Haloperidol is a butyrophenone antipsychotic agent that is available as tablets and an oral solution.

Mechanism of Toxicity: Haloperidol administration results in decreased levels of brain catecholamines, presumably by preventing reuptake at synaptic terminals. Haloperidol also appears to antagonize brain dopamine action and lowers the seizure threshold. Anticholinergic effects are less prominent with haloperidol than with phenothiazine antipsychotics. Antidopaminergic effects are believed to contribute to acute dystonic reactions, extrapyramidal symptoms, catatonic syndromes, and neuroleptic malignant syndrome, which have been reported after therapeutic doses or overdose.

Toxic Dose: Some adverse effects of haloperidol may occur at a therapeutic dose, which in children is about 0.05 mg/kg/d. A toxic dose in children is not defined, although no deaths have been reported. Ingestion of other central nervous system depressants with haloperidol may potentiate its sedative effects. Because haloperidol has a long elimination half-life (about 21 hours), dystonic reactions may recur for up to 5 to 7 days after the last dose.

Signs and Symptoms: Following acute overdose, haloperidol produces central nervous system depression with lethargy, coma, and decreased respiratory effort. Hypothermia and hypotension may be present.

Acute dystonic reactions are more common in children younger than 15 years. Symptoms include torticollis, oculogyric crisis, and opisthotonos. These reactions may be mistaken for a seizure, and patients have been described as appearing to be awake but having a seizure. Extrapyramidal symptoms include facial grimacing and muscle rigidity, dysarthria, dysphonia, and cogwheel rigidity of the extremities.

The triad of hyperthermia, altered mentation (eg, confusion, stupor, or decreased alertness), and muscle rigidity are pathognomonic for neuroleptic malignant syndrome. Temperatures can be as high as 107°F. Patients with neuroleptic malignant syndrome have autonomic instability (labile hypertension, tachycardia, sweating, pallor, and vasoconstriction) and rapidly develop lactic acidosis, rhabdomyolysis, hypocalcemia, electrolyte imbalance, hypoxia, and seizures. The occurrence of seizures in a hyperthermic patient with neuroleptic malignant syndrome is associated with a high risk for permanent central nervous system damage.

Diagnostic Testing: Haloperidol may be detected in drug screens. Serum levels are not clinically available or useful.

General Treatment: Because significant symptoms are possible, the need for life support measures including respiratory support and cardiac monitoring should be anticipated.

Decontamination: (Refer to the treatment section p 6 for the appropriate use of these techniques.) Gastric lavage is the preferred method of gastric emptying if the ingestion is recent (<2 hours). Emesis is not recommended if lethargy, dysarthria, or muscle dysfunction is present because of the potential for aspiration. Activated charcoal can be used with or in place of gastric lavage.

Antidote: No specific antidotes are available.

Specific Treatment: (See Table 2, p 16, for specific dosing.)
Acute dystonic reactions and extrapyramidal symptoms can be treated with intravenous diphenhydramine or benztropine (Cogentin). Once acute symptoms resolve, oral therapy with diphenhydramine (every 6 hours) or benztropine (every 12 hours) should be continued for 5 to 6 days to prevent recurrence of symptoms.

Neuroleptic malignant syndrome is a medical emergency that requires aggressive measures to reduce body temperature (ie, cooling blanket, iced saline gastric lavage, cooled intravenous fluids). Antipyretics are ineffective and contraindicated. Endotracheal intubation is needed to ventilate the patient adequately. Intravenous fluids should be used for cooling, to correct dehydration, and to maintain urine flow, which may prevent myoglobin-induced renal failure. Dantrolene (see Table 3, p 22, for specific dosing) may be effective in relaxing muscle rigidity, and, if used, it should be continued for 5 days. The drug can be given orally once the patient can tolerate oral intake. Diazepam has also been effective for muscle relaxation in some individuals. Bromocriptine is a dopamine agonist that has reversed hyperpyrexia and muscle rigidity when used in adults at doses of 5 to 7.5 mg every 8 hours. Treat acidosis with bicarbonate. Seizures must be managed aggressively with benzodiazepines.

Patient Monitoring: If neuroleptic malignant syndrome is suspected, obtain arterial blood gases, serum electrolytes, calcium, creatine phosphokinase, liver function tests, and monitor urine for myoglobin and output.

Enhanced Elimination: Enhanced elimination techniques are of no proven value.

References

Hoffman AS, Schwartz HI, Novick RM. Catatonic reaction to accidental haloperidol overdose: an unrecognized drug abuse risk. *J Nerv Ment Dis.* 1986;174:428-430

Joshi PT, Capozzoli JA, Coyle JT. Neuroleptic malignant syndrome: life threatening complication of neuroleptic treatment in adolescents with affective disorder. *Pediatrics*. 1991;87:235-239

Knight ME, Roberts RJ. Phenothiazine and butyrophenone intoxication in children. *Pediatr Clin North Am*. 1986;33:299-309

Nierenberg D, Disch M, Manheimer E, et al. Facilitating prompt diagnosis and treatment of the neuroleptic malignant syndrome. *Clin Pharmacol Ther*. 1991;50:580-586

Schneider SM. Neuroleptic malignant syndrome: controversies in treatment. *Am J Emerg Med*. 1991;9:360-362

Scialli JV, Thornton WE. Toxic reactions from a haloperidol overdose in two children: thermal and cardiac manifestations. *JAMA*. 1978;239:48-49

Sinaniotis CA, Spyrides P, Vlachos P, Papadatos C. Acute haloperidol poisoning in children. *J Pediatr*. 1978;93:1038-1039

Hypoglycemic Agents — Oral

Available Forms and Sources: See Table 10 for available hypoglycemic agents.

Mechanism of Toxicity: The hypoglycemic action of these agents occurs in both diabetic and nondiabetic individuals. The mechanism of action is incompletely understood, but the major effect appears to be the stimulation of insulin secretion. Additionally, oral hypoglycemic agents appear to have extrapancreatic actions including enhancing peripheral sensitivity to circulating insulin and reduced hepatic glucose production. Because oral hypoglycemic agents contain a sulphur nucleus, allergic reactions have been reported in those with sulfonamide allergies.

Toxic Dose: The toxic dose varies with each compound. Doses of glyburide as low as 10 to 15 mg have caused severe hypoglycemia in children.

Signs and Symptoms: Plasma levels of oral hypoglycemic agents peak within 1 to 8 hours of ingestion, resulting in the prompt appearance of symptoms. Manifestations include hypoglycemia with secondary coma and seizures. Prolonged hypoglycemia may be resistant to treatment and may cause

Table 10. Available Oral Hypoglycemic Agents*

Drug	Dosage, Strengths, mg	Relative Potency	Duration of Action, h
Tolbutamide (Orinase)	250, 500	1	6-10
Acetohexamide (Dymelor)	250, 500	2.5	12-18
Tolazamide (Tolinase)	100, 250, 500	5	16-24
Chlorpropamide (Diabinese)	100, 250	6	24-72
Glipizide (Glucotrol)	5, 10	100	16-24
Glyburide (Diabeta, Micronase, Glynase)	1.25, 2.5, 3, 5	150	18-24

*Adapted from Oates and Wood.

permanent cerebral injury. Other reported toxic reactions include inappropriate antidiuretic hormone secretion with severe hyponatremia. Metabolic acidosis may also occur. Hypotension, tachycardia, and cardiac arrest have been reported in severe cases.

Diagnostic Testing: These agents generally are not detected by a routine drug screen. Specific measurements of serum drug concentrations are difficult to obtain and are not clinically useful.

General Treatment: Because significant symptoms are possible, the need for life support measures should be anticipated.

Decontamination: (Refer to the treatment section p 6 for the appropriate use of these techniques.) Emesis can be used if instituted early after the ingestion. Gastric lavage with activated charcoal or activated charcoal alone may also be used.

Antidote: (See Table 2, p 16, for specific dosing.) Severe hypoglycemia is initially treated with intravenous administration of a 20% to 50% glucose solution. Glucagon may be administered intravenously or intramuscularly, although it typically has little effectiveness in reversing the hypoglycemia induced by oral hypoglycemic agents. The antihypertensive diazoxide is a potent hyperglycemic agent that inhibits insulin secretion and increases hepatic release of glucose.

Specific Treatment: Seizures can be treated with benzodiazepines, phenytoin, or both. Close monitoring of blood pressure is necessary because of the risk of significant hypotension. All patients who develop hypoglycemia should be admitted to the hospital for close monitoring of serum glucose levels. Because of the risk of recurrent hypoglycemia and reports of deaths occurring more than 24 hours after ingestion, observation for at least 24 hours after resolution of symptoms is recommended.

Patient Monitoring: Electrolyte levels, arterial blood gases, and serial measurements of blood glucose should be monitored.

Enhanced Elimination: Enhanced elimination techniques are of no proven value.

References

Erickson T, Arora A, Lebby TI, Lipscomp JW, Leikin JB. Acute oral hypoglycemic ingestions. *Vet Hum Toxicol.* 1991;33:256-258

Gerich JE. Oral hypoglycemic agents. *N Engl J Med.* 1989;321:1231-1245

Ibuprofen

Available Forms and Sources: This nonsteroidal anti-inflammatory agent is available over-the-counter and by prescription. It is formulated as a single agent in tablets, caplets, and a pediatric suspension. It is also formulated as an ingredient in many cough and cold preparations. Trade names for ibuprofen include Motrin and Advil.

Mechanism of Toxicity: Ibuprofen inhibits prostaglandin synthesis, which is the likely mechanism for its gastrointestinal effects. The mechanism of action for the central nervous system effects is not elucidated.

Toxic Dose: Acute ingestions of ≤100 mg/kg are usually well tolerated. Ingestions of >300 mg/kg are associated with an increased incidence of significant signs and symptoms.

Signs and Symptoms: Nausea, vomiting, and abdominal pain are common symptoms even following minor ingestions. Commonly reported central nervous system effects include lethargy, drowsiness, and tinnitus. Apnea, coma, and seizures have been reported following exposures of >400 mg/kg. Transient acute renal failure is uncommon. An elevated anion gap metabolic acidosis can occur following large ingestions. Hypokalemia has been reported.

Diagnostic Testing: Ibuprofen can be qualitatively detected by most drug screening techniques. Serum ibuprofen levels may provide some prognostic value to assess the severity of the exposure; however, the correlation between blood levels and symptoms has been disputed. Serum levels generally are not available.

General Treatment: Significant acute symptoms are not anticipated following ingestions of ≤100 mg/kg. Administer fluids or food to minimize gastrointestinal upset.

Decontamination: (Refer to the treatment section p 6 for the appropriate use of these techniques.) Emesis at home may be safely used if 100 to 300 mg/kg has been ingested. Treatment with emesis, lavage, or activated charcoal in a health care facility should be considered if >300 mg/kg has been ingested.

Antidote: No specific antidotes are available.

Specific Treatment: Treat hypokalemia and metabolic acidosis as needed, and treat seizures using the standard anticonvulsants. Support respiration as needed.

Patient Monitoring: Obtain levels of electrolytes, arterial blood gases, and perform renal function tests following significant exposures.

Enhanced Elimination: Enhanced elimination techniques are of no proven value.

References

Hall AH, Smolinske SC, Conrad FL, et al. Ibuprofen overdose: 126 cases. *Ann Emerg Med.*1986;11:1308-1313

McElwee NE, Veltri JC, Bradford DC, Rollins DE. A prospective, population-based study of acute ibuprofen overdose: complications are rare and routine serum levels not warranted. *Ann Emerg Med.*1990;19:657-662

Imidazoles
(Nose and Eye Drops)

Available Forms and Sources: Three imidazole compounds —oxymetazoline, naphazoline, and tetrahydrozoline—are used topically for long-acting vasoconstriction. They are sold as nasal sprays in a 0.1% concentration and as eye drops in a 0.05% concentration. Common product names include Afrin, Duration-12, Vicks Sinex Long-acting, Murine, Visine, and Privine.

Mechanism of Toxicity: These compounds are peripheral and central α-adrenergic agonists that decrease central sympathetic outflow.

Toxic Dose: Infants may be sedated following the instillation of a drop or two of the nasal products. Ingestion of 3.5 mg has led to obtundation. A 15-mL bottle of 0.1% drug contains 15 mg, so the ingestion of any amount should be considered potentially toxic to a 2-year-old child. Adverse reactions to oxymetazoline nose drops have been reported in children (aged 5 weeks to 5 years) at recommended doses.

Signs and Symptoms: Seizures, drowsiness, tachycardia, hypothermia, excitation, miosis, and hallucinations have been reported, which resolve over 24 hours. Excess use late in pregnancy has led to late decelerations in the heart rate of the infant in utero.

Diagnostic Testing: These agents are not identified in routine drug screens. They may cause false-positive results in immunoassay screening tests for cannabinoids.

General Treatment: Life-threatening acute symptoms are not anticipated. Patients should be evaluated and supportive care provided as needed.

Decontamination: (Refer to the treatment section p 6 for the appropriate use of these techniques.) Emesis is contraindicated because of the rapid onset of central nervous system depression. Because of the small volumes and rapid absorption of these agents, gastric lavage is of questionable value. Activated charcoal may be administered following large ingestions if instituted early.

Antidote: α-Adrenergic antagonists (eg, tolazoline) are rarely required.

Specific Treatment: Seizures can be treated with standard anticonvulsant agents.

Patient Monitoring: Monitor ventilation and perfusion until the patient is awake.

Enhanced Elimination: Enhanced elimination techniques are of no proven value.

References

Baxi LV, Gindoff PR, Pregenzer GJ, Parras MK. Fetal heart rate changes following maternal administration of a nasal decongestant. *Am J Obstet Gynecol.* 1985;153:799-800

Klein-Schwartz W, Gorman R, Oderda GM, Baig A. Central nervous system depression from ingestion of nonprescription eyedrops. *Am J Emerg Med.* 1984;2:217-218

Mikkelsen SL, Ash KO. Adulterants causing false negatives in illicit drug testing. *Clin Chem.* 1988;34:2333-2336

Söderman P, Sahlberg D, Wiholm BE. Central nervous system reactions to nose drops in small children. *Lancet.* 1984;1:573

Iron

Available Forms and Sources: Iron preparations usually contain one of three ferrous salts—either sulfate, fumarate, or gluconate. They are available in both over-the-counter and prescription preparations as a single agent and in combination with other vitamins and minerals. Formulations include tablets, chewable tablets, capsules, and liquids.

Mechanism of Toxicity: Ferrous iron is absorbed into the mucosal cells of the duodenum and jejunum and oxidized to ferric iron, where it is bound to ferritin, an iron storage protein. It is then released from ferritin into the plasma, where it is bound to transferrin, an iron-specific binding globulin. Iron bound to transferrin is nontoxic. Excess free iron (iron exceeding the iron-binding capacity) is directly toxic to the vasculature and also leads to the release of vasoactive substances including serotonin and histamine. Excess quantities of ferritin result in vasodilation. These mechanisms result in increased vascular permeability and fluid loss, with subsequent hypotension and metabolic acidosis. In overdose, iron is deposited in the liver, spleen, and kidneys. Fatty degeneration and necrosis are seen in hepatocytes, renal tubules, and myocardial cells.

Toxic Dose: Toxicity is dependent on the amount of elemental iron available in the various salt forms (20% for sulfate, 33% for fumarate, and 12% for gluconate). Ingestion of more than 20 mg/kg of elemental iron produces gastrointestinal effects, ingestion of more than 60 mg/kg causes systemic toxic effects, and ingestion of more than 250 mg/kg is potentially lethal.

Signs and Symptoms: Acute iron poisoning in children characteristically follows a biphasic course. Vomiting usually occurs within 30 minutes to 1 hour after ingestion. Vomitus may be bloody, contain partially digested tablets, and may continue for several hours. Enteric-coated tablets may pass into the small intestine without causing gastric symptoms. Abdominal cramps, tarry stools or bloody diarrhea, lethargy, and, in severe cases, acidosis and shock may occur within the first 6 to 12 hours. Leukocytosis and fever may also be present. The child may appear to improve clinically after this first phase, then unexpectedly may experience profound cardiovascular collapse hours later. This second phase is often associated with hepatic injury. The latent period between these two symptomatic phases may last several hours. The course is difficult to predict. Late complications developing several weeks to months after exposure include hepatic cirrhosis and pyloric or duodenal stenosis.

Diagnostic Testing: Iron is not detected on a routine drug screen. A serum iron level should be obtained within 4 to 6 hours of ingestion. If available, a total iron-binding capacity should be determined 2 to 4 hours after ingestion. Gastrointestinal symptoms may occur with iron levels that are less than the iron binding capacity (<300 μg/dL). Some patients experience symptoms with an iron level between 300 and 500 μg/dL. Serum iron levels >1000 μg/dL are considered potentially lethal. When the ingestion of iron is uncertain but may have occurred within the preceding 4 hours, the deferoxamine color test may be helpful for determining the presence of iron in gastric contents (hydrogen peroxide and deferoxamine added to gastric contents turn the gastric aspirate a vin rosé color).

General Treatment: Significant acute symptoms are not anticipated. General supportive care should be provided as required.

Decontamination: (Refer to the treatment section p 6 for the appropriate use of these techniques.) Emesis may be more effective than gastric lavage because it is difficult to remove the large iron tablets through a tube. If tablets are not removed by emesis, they may need to be removed from the stomach with whole bowel irrigation. Endoscopic or surgical removal should be used only in extreme cases. Activated charcoal does not bind iron. Lavage with a 5% sodium bicarbonate solution can be performed with 100 mL of the solution left in the stomach to convert any free ferrous salt to insoluble ferrous carbonate, thereby reducing iron absorption as well as the local irritative effects of iron. A disodium phosphate solution (Fleet enema) also has been used instead of sodium bicarbonate, but hypocalcemia with seizures has occurred. There are no data to suggest that phosphate is more effective than bicarbonate, and therefore its use should be avoided. All treated patients should be seen within 2 weeks of discharge to ensure that there are no gastrointestinal sequelae.

Antidote: Deferoxamine (Desferal) is a specific chelating agent for iron (see **Table 2, p 16, for specific dosing**). Indications for deferoxamine include patients with serum iron levels of ≥500 µg/dL, with or without symptoms, and patients with significant symptoms of hypotension, and acidosis regardless of the serum iron level. The iron-ferroxamine complex produces an orange-rose or vin rosé color in the patient's urine.

The use of oral deferoxamine is controversial. In studies using dogs it effectively binds iron in the gastrointestinal tract, and although the iron-deferoxamine complex (ferrioxamine) is absorbed it appears to exhibit low toxicity. The cost and questionable efficacy preclude its routine use.

Specific Treatment: If metabolic acidosis is present, sodium bicarbonate should be administered in an intravenous line separate from deferoxamine. Shock may require intensive supportive therapy. Blood replacement, plasma replacement, or both may be necessary. Antacids can be administered to protect the upper gastrointestinal tract.

Patient Monitoring: Iron tablets (but not multivitamins with iron) in the stomach or small bowel are visible on roentgenogram. All stools and emesis should be tested for blood. Roentgenographic or barium swallow examinations of the gastrointestinal tract may be indicated if stricture is suspected. Monitor the patient for iron deficiency from blood loss and excessive chelation therapy.

Enhanced Elimination: Enhanced elimination techniques are of no proven value to remove iron. The iron-ferrioxamine complex is removed by dialysis.

References

Henretig FM, Temple AR. Acute poisoning in children. *Emerg Med Clin North Am.* 1984;2:121-132

Jacobs J, Greene H, Gendel BR. Acute iron intoxication. *N Engl J Med.* 1965;273:1124-1127

Lacouture PG, Wason S, Temple AR, Wallace DK, Lovejoy FH Jr. Emergency assessment of severity in iron overdose by clinical and laboratory methods. *J Pediatr.* 1981;99:89-91

McGuigan MA, Lovejoy FH Jr, Marino SK, Propper RD, Goldman P. Qualitative deferoxamine color test for iron ingestion. *J Pediatr.* 1979; 94:940-942

Proudfoot AT, Simpson D, Dyson EH. Management of acute iron poisoning. *Med Toxicol.* 1986;1:83-100

Robotham JL, Lietman PS. Acute iron poisoning—a review. *AJDC.* 1980; 134:875-879

Isoniazid (INH)

Available Forms and Sources: Isoniazid (INH), used in the treatment of tuberculosis, is available in tablets, a syrup, and an injectable form.

Mechanism of Toxicity: Isoniazid produces acute toxic effects by competing with pyridoxal 5-phosphate (the active form of vitamin B_6) in the central nervous system for the enzyme glutamic acid decarboxylase (GABA), which is an inhibitory neurotransmitter in the brain. A decrease in GABA levels can lead to uninhibited electrical activity that manifests as seizures. Isoniazid also inhibits the conversion of lactate to pyruvate, resulting in lactic acidosis.

Toxic Dose: A dose of 15 mg/kg can lower the seizure threshold; 35 to 40 mg/kg can induce spontaneous seizures.

Signs and Symptoms: The typical clinical picture consists of repetitive seizures, metabolic acidosis, and coma. Initial clinical signs include nausea, vomiting, blurred vision, ataxia, increased deep tendon reflexes, hyperthermia, and tachycardia. Often a latent period of 30 to 120 minutes occurs before abnormal signs and symptoms appear. A severe anion gap metabolic acidosis can develop following only one or two seizures.

Diagnostic Testing: Isoniazid is not detected in routine drug screens, and serum levels are generally not available. Therapeutic levels range from 5 to 8 µg/mL. Acute toxic levels exceed 20 µg/mL.

General Treatment: Because significant symptoms are possible, the need for life support measures including respiratory support should be anticipated.

Decontamination: (Refer to the treatment section p 6 for the appropriate use of these techniques.) Emesis is not recommended because of the risk of seizures. Gastric lavage may be helpful if instituted soon after the ingestion. Activated charcoal can be used with a cathartic.

Antidote: Pyridoxine hydrochloride given intravenously is a specific antidote for INH-induced seizures and usually stops seizures resistant to diazepam treatment. Pyridoxine should be administered until the seizures are well controlled (see Table 2, p 16, for specific dosing).

Specific Treatment: (See Tables 2 and 3, pp 16 and 22, respectively, for specific dosing.) Seizures can be treated with intravenous diazepam; pyridoxine, however, is the agent of choice. Acidosis is treated with sodium bicarbonate. Provide aggressive supportive care.

Patient Monitoring: Monitor acid-base balance and electrolytes.

Enhanced Elimination: Peritoneal or hemodialysis may remove the drug, but should be reserved for those patients unresponsive to therapy using anticonvulsants, pyridoxine, and bicarbonate.

References

Black LE, Ros SP. Complete recovery from severe metabolic acidosis associated with isoniazid poisoning in a young boy. *Pediatr Emerg Care.* 1989;5:257-258

Brown A, Mallett M, Fiser D, Arnold WC. Acute isoniazid intoxication: reversal of central nervous system symptoms with large doses of pyridoxine. *Pediatr Pharmacol.* 1984;4:199-202

Miller J, Robinson A, Percy AK. Acute isoniazid poisoning in childhood. *AJDC*. 1980;134:290

Siefkin AD, Albertson TE, Corbett MG. Isoniazid overdose: pharma-cokinetics and effects of oral charcoal in treatment. *Hum Toxicol*. 1987; 6:497-501

Laxatives

Available Forms and Sources: Bulk-forming laxatives include psyllium and polycarbophil. Emollient types of laxatives include mineral oil, docusate calcium (Surfak), and docusate sodium (Colace). Saline types of laxatives include magnesium sulfate (Epsom salt), magnesium citrate, sodium sulfate, and sodium phosphate. Irritant types of laxatives include phenol-phthalein, castor oil, cascara sagrada, bisacodyl, and senna. Osmotic types of laxatives include sorbitol and glycerin.

Mechanism of Toxicity: The mechanism of toxicity for these agents is an extension of their pharmacologic actions.

Toxic Dose: The toxic dose for most of these agents is not defined. Doses of phenolphthalein as high as 1 g have produced only mild symptoms.

Signs and Symptoms: Acute exposure to most laxatives pro-duces nausea, vomiting, and diarrhea, which are usually mild and self-limiting. Significant fluid loss and dehydration are uncom-mon. Magnesium toxicity with muscle weakness and central nervous system depression usually develops only after a single massive or long-term exposure. Hypersensitivity reactions to phenolphthalein have been reported but are rare. Phenolphthalein may also produce abdominal cramps and a pink to red discolora-tion of urine and feces. Emollient agents, particularly mineral oil, can cause aspiration pneumonitis (see hydrocarbon manage-ment, p 194).

Diagnostic Testing: None of these agents are detected on routine drug screens. Alkalinization of 10 mL of urine with 2 mL of 0.1N sodium hydroxide produces a pink color if phenolphthalein is present.

General Treatment: Significant acute symptoms are not anticipated. After a single severe exposure, observation and fluid replacement, if necessary, is usually the only treatment required.

Decontamination: (Refer to the treatment section p 6 for the appropriate use of these techniques.) Emesis is contraindicated following the ingestion of emollient-type agents. Following the ingestion of irritants, emesis can be used if instituted early. Activated charcoal alone may also be used. Cathartics should not be used.

Antidote: No specific antidotes are available.

Specific Treatment: Treatment is supportive. There is no specific treatment.

Patient Monitoring: Levels of electrolytes should be monitored following significant exposures. Serum magnesium levels should be monitored following significant exposures to magnesium-containing saline cathartics.

Enhanced Elimination: Hemodialysis may be used to treat hypermagnesemia following the administration of saline cathartics.

References

Buchanan N, Cane RD, Glantz R, Hunt JA. Phenophthalien poisoning: a case report. *S Afr Med J.* 1976;50:1060

de Oliveira GA, Del Caro SR, Bender-Lamego CM, Mercon-de-Vargas PR, Vervloet VE. Radiographic plain film and CT findings in lipoid pneumonia in infants following aspiration of mineral oil used in the treatment of partial small bowel obstruction by *Ascaris lumbricoides. Pediatr Radiol.* 1985;15:157-160

Devore CD, Ulshen MH, Cross RE. Phenophthalien laxatives and factitious diarrhea. *Clin Pediatr.* 1982;21:573-574

Larson JE, Swigart SA, Angle CR. Laxative phosphate poisoning: pharmacokinetics of serum phosphorous. *Hum Toxicol.* 1986;5:45-49

Lithium

Available Forms and Sources: Lithium is available as a carbonate or citrate salt. Product formulations include tablets, capsules, liquids, and sustained-release preparations. Lithium is also used industrially in batteries, alloys, and lubricating greases.

Mechanism of Toxicity: Lithium is thought to interfere with physiologic processes involving other monovalent cations such as sodium and potassium.

Toxic Dose: Significant toxicity from a single severe ingestion is unlikely in patients not currently being treated with lithium. However, even small overdoses in patients receiving long-term therapy are potentially toxic.

One gram of lithium carbonate contains 189 mg of lithium. It is estimated that each 300-mg dose of lithium increases serum lithium levels by 0.2 to 0.4 mEq/L.

Signs and Symptoms: After an acute overdose, nausea, vomiting, and diarrhea may develop. Acute overdose in patients receiving long-term lithium therapy may also present with these signs and symptoms. Neurologic effects such as tremor, slurred speech, lethargy, and decreased level of consciousness also occur as can cardiac conduction disturbances. Cardiac dysrhythmias may occur; particularly in comatose patients.

Diagnostic Testing: Lithium is not detected in most routine drug screens. Lithium levels, however, are routinely determined in most laboratories. In patients who have not taken lithium previously, serial lithium serum concentrations should be obtained only after large ingestions. In patients receiving long-term lithium therapy, serial serum lithium levels should be obtained even though the correlation of levels with the degree of clinical toxicity is not great. Therapeutic levels are 0.6 to 1.2 mEq/L, with severe intoxication seen at levels >2.5 mEq/L. Levels should be monitored closely in patients receiving long-term lithium therapy.

General Treatment: Because significant symptoms are possible, the need for life support measures including cardiovascular monitoring should be anticipated.

Decontamination: (Refer to the treatment section p 6 for the appropriate use of these techniques.) Emesis is of value following recent ingestions. Activated charcoal does not adsorb lithium. Whole bowel irrigation is the procedure of choice, especially if a delayed-release formulation is involved.

Antidote: No specific antidotes are available.

Specific Treatment: Treatment is generally supportive. There is no specific treatment.

Patient Monitoring: Levels of serum electrolytes should be monitored.

Enhanced Elimination: Saline diuresis enhances the renal clearance of lithium. Hemodialysis effectively removes lithium and should be considered in symptomatic patients with serum concentrations >2.5 mEq/L.

References

Goetting MG. Acute lithium poisoning in a child with dystonia. *Pediatrics.* 1985;76:978-980

Smith SW, Ling LJ, Halstenson CE. Whole-bowel irrigation as a treatment for acute lithium overdose. *Ann Emerg Med.* 1991;20:536-539

Local Anesthetics

Available Forms and Sources: Agents included in this group include benzocaine, procaine, chloroprocaine, tetracaine, bupivacaine, prilocaine, lidocaine, etidocaine, and mepivacaine. Cocaine is discussed in a separate chapter (p 143).

Mechanism of Toxicity: Local anesthetics exert their pharmacologic and toxicologic effects by blocking sodium channels in peripheral and central nerve fibers, thus slowing or blocking impulse generation. Benzocaine and lidocaine can also produce methemoglobinemia following ingestion in infants.

Toxic Dose: A toxic dose for these agents is not well defined. Accidental intravenous injection of doses intended for local wound infiltration has resulted in seizures, cardiac dysrhythmias, and death.

Ingestion of 5 to 30 mL of 2% viscous lidocaine has produced seizures in children. Topical application of 2% viscous lidocaine to the gums, five to six times per day, has also been reported to cause seizures. Toxic reactions also have been reported in infants born of mothers receiving local anesthesia for pudendal block.

Signs and Symptoms: The primary target organ of local anesthetic poisoning is the central nervous system. Observed signs and symptoms include headache, slurred speech, anxiety, confusion, perioral paresthesias, tinnitus, miosis, seizures, and coma. Cardiac dysrhythmias associated with hypotension may also occur. Asystole has been seen following inadvertent intravenous injection of local anesthetics.

Diagnostic Testing: Local anesthetics can be detected in blood and urine and are detected by most routine drug screens. Quantitation of serum lidocaine may be useful in assessing the toxicity of this agent. Quantitation of the other agents is not clinically useful. Cyanosis due to methemoglobinemia can be seen in infants after lidocaine and benzocaine ingestion.

General Treatment: Because significant symptoms are possible, the need for life support measures including cardiorespiratory support should be anticipated following significant exposures.

Decontamination: (Refer to the treatment section p 6 for the appropriate use of these techniques.) Emesis should be avoided. Treatment with activated charcoal and gastric lavage should be considered if instituted early after the exposure.

Antidote: No specific antidotes are available.

Specific Treatment: Treatment is symptomatic only.

Patient Monitoring: After ingestion of large quantities of benzocaine or lidocaine, methemoglobin levels should be monitored.

Enhanced Elimination: Forced diuresis has been reported to increase the clearance of mepivacaine. In general, enhanced elimination is not of value.

References

Amitai Y, Whitesell L, Lovejoy FH. Death following accidental lidocaine overdose in a child. *N Engl J Med.* 1986;314:182-183

Bozynski ME, Rubarth LB, Patel JA. Lidocaine toxicity after maternal pudendal anesthesia in a term infant with fetal distress. *Am J Perinatol.* 1987;4:164-166

Mofenson HC, Caraccio TR, Miller H, Greensher J. Lidocaine toxicity from topical mucosal application: with a review of the clinical pharmacology of lidocaine. *Clin Pediatr.* 1983;22:190-192

Lomotil

Available Forms and Sources: Diphenoxylate-atropine (Lomotil) is available in a fixed combination that contains 2.5 mg of diphenoxylate and 0.025 mg of atropine sulfate per tablet or 5-mL of liquid.

Mechanism of Toxicity: Atropine is a potent anticholinergic drug whose pharmacologic effect is competitive inhibition of postsynaptic, muscarinic (cholinergic) receptors. Diphenoxylate is a semisynthetic opiate that produces classic manifestations of narcotic overdose (ie, central nervous system depression). Diphenoxylate is metabolized to difenoxin, an active product that may be responsible for the recurrent respiratory depression that often accompanies an overdose of Lomotil.

Toxic Dose: Manifestations of Lomotil toxicity can appear with ingestion of one tablet in a child. Ingestion of two tablets invariably leads to clinical manifestations. Death has been reported after ingestion of a single tablet in a 2-year-old, although fatalities in children are more typically associated with ingestions of 10 to 15 tablets.

Signs and Symptoms: Clinical signs of toxicity appear within 1 to 4 hours after ingestion. Although traditionally Lomotil ingestion was thought to cause biphasic intoxication, with atropine-induced anticholinergic effects appearing early (within 2 to 3 hours of ingestion) and symptoms of opiate toxicity appearing late, more recent data suggest that signs of opiate intoxication may precede signs of atropinism, or both may appear simultaneously. Anticholinergic effects typically last up to 12 hours. Signs of atropinism include hyperpyrexia, flushed skin, dry mucous membranes, and tachycardia. Signs of opiate intoxication include respiratory depression and miosis. With severe toxicity cardiac arrest may occur. Flaccidity may also occur. Recurrent opiate-induced central nervous system depression may continue for 6 to 24 hours after ingestion. Paralytic ileus may develop.

Diagnostic Testing: Diphenoxylate and atropine are detected by most routine drug screens. The measurement of atropine or diphenoxylate levels in serum or urine is not clinically useful.

General Treatment: All children who have ingested Lomotil must be admitted to the hospital for 24 hours of observation because of the risk of recurrent respiratory depression.

Decontamination: (Refer to the treatment section p 6 for the appropriate use of these techniques.) Emesis is contraindicated because of the risk of central nervous system and respiratory depression, which may occur within 1 hour of ingestion. Gastric lavage may be effective for several hours after ingestion. Activated charcoal with a dose of cathartic should be administered unless bowel sounds are absent.

Antidote: Naloxone is highly effective in reversing opiate-induced central nervous system depression. In cases of severe intoxication, a continuous naloxone infusion may be necessary to sustain its effect. Physostigmine may reverse the anticholinergic effects of atropine, but because of its associated hazards (severe bradycardia and seizures) it is not recommended (see Table 2, p 16, for specific dosing).

Specific Treatment: Cardiac disturbances, which consist primarily of tachydysrhythmias, may require the use of antidysrhythmics or cardioversion. Other care is symptomatic.

Patient Monitoring: Blood gases should be monitored in patients with respiratory depression.

Enhanced Elimination: The elimination of difenoxin is potentially enhanced by the administration of multiple-dose activated charcoal. Repeated doses of activated charcoal should not be administered if bowel sounds are absent.

References

Curtis JA, Goel KM. Lomotil poisoning in children. *Arch Dis Child.* 1979;54:222-225

McCarron MM, Challoner KR, Thompson GA. Diphenoxylate-atropine (Lomotil) overdose in children: an update (report of eight cases and review of the literature). *Pediatrics.* 1991;87:694-700

Rumack BH, Temple AR. Lomotil poisoning. *Pediatrics.* 1974;53:495-500

Wasserman GS. Lomotil overdose. *Pediatrics.* 1991;88:1294-1295

Loperamide

Available Forms and Sources: Loperamide is an antidiarrheal agent that is available as a prescription and over-the-counter drug (Imodium A-D).

Mechanism of Toxicity: Loperamide has a chemical structure similar to that of haloperidol and diphenoxylate (Lomotil). The toxicity of loperamide is likely to be the result of its opioid-like activity.

Toxic Dose: Changes in personality have been reported after doses of 0.1 to 0.12 mg/kg/d in toddlers. Doses of 0.1 to 2.0 mg/kg have caused respiratory and central nervous system depression. It has been speculated that children are more susceptible to the toxic effects than adults. Several deaths have been reported following complications secondary to loperamide misuse in children younger than 7 months.

Signs and Symptoms: The clinical picture is the classic narcotic triad of coma, miosis, and respiratory depression. Miosis is a common finding but may be absent if hypoxia, severe acidosis, or severe respiratory depression is present. Respiratory depression can progress to respiratory acidosis and apnea. Central nervous system disturbances include irritability, personality changes, varying degrees of central nervous system depression, and seizures. Other possible signs include bradycardia and paralytic ileus. Because the chemical structure of loperamide is similar to haloperidol, acute dystonic reactions are possible but rare.

Diagnostic Testing: Loperamide is detected on routine drug screens. The quantitation of serum levels is not clinically useful.

General Treatment: Because significant symptoms are possible, the need for life support measures including respiratory and cardiovascular support should be anticipated.

Decontamination: (Refer to the treatment section p 6 for the appropriate use of these techniques.) Emesis is contraindicated because of the rapid onset of central nervous system depression and seizures. Activated charcoal may be administered.

Antidote: Naloxone can be given intermittently and repeated as needed or can be given as a continuous infusion. Dystonic reactions can be treated with intravenous benztropine (Cogentin) or diphenhydramine (see Table 2, p 16, for specific dosing).

Specific Treatment: Mechanical ventilation may be needed if ventilation cannot be maintained with naloxone. Other treatment is routine and symptomatic.

Patient Monitoring: Blood gases should be monitored if the respiratory status of the patient is compromised.

Enhanced Elimination: Enhanced elimination techniques are of no proven value.

References

Bhutta TI, Tahir KI. Loperamide poisoning in children. *Lancet.* 1990;335:363

Minton NA, Smith PG. Loperamide toxicity in a child after a single dose. *Br Med J.* 1987;294:1303

Tan SH. Loperamide toxicity in an infant. *Aust Paediatr J.* 1983;19:55

MAO Inhibitors

Available Forms and Sources: Isocarboxazid (Marplan), phenelzine (Nardil), and tranylcypromine (Parnate) are monoamine oxidase inhibitors (MAO inhibitors) used primarily for the treatment of depression. Selegiline (Eldepryl) is used as an adjunct for the treatment of Parkinson's disease.

Mechanism of Toxicity: Monoamine oxidase inhibitors (MAOI) act by permanently inhibiting the activity of the enzyme monoamine oxidase. In the absence of this enzyme, which is responsible for the inactivation of catecholamines, the actions of all biogenic amines, both endogenous and exogenous, are potentiated.

Three distinct syndromes can appear in association with MAO inhibitor toxicity.

Biogenic amine interaction. Many amines in foods and medications act as indirect sympathomimetics, stimulating the release of endogenous catecholamines from presynaptic nerve terminals (Tables 11 and 12). Monoamine oxidase in the gastrointestinal tract typically inactivates these amines before their systemic absorption. With inhibition of the enzyme by MAO inhibitors, these amines may be absorbed, leading to massive release of endogenous catecholamines.

Opioid hyperserotonergic interaction. Administration of certain agents, particularly meperidine and, to a lesser extent, dextromethorphan, has been associated with the abrupt appearance of hyperserotonergic effects including agitation and hyperpyrexia.

Overdose. A single massive overdose of MAO inhibitors alone is associated with the sometimes delayed appearance of an adrenergic crisis.

Table 11. Significant Drug Interactions With Monoamine Oxidase Inhibitors*

Absolutely Contraindicated	Avoid
Ephedrine	Other narcotics
Phenylephrine	Dextromethorphan
Phenylpropanolamine	Reserpine
Metaraminol	Guanethidine
Amphetamines	Atropine
Cocaine	Thiazide diuretics
Meperidine	Direct sympathomimetics
L-Dopa	

*Adapted from Haddad and Winchester

Table 12. Significant Food Interactions With Monoamine Oxidase Inhibitors*

Any high-protein food that has undergone aging, fermentation, pickling, smoking, or bacterial contamination

Aged cheese

Decayed or spoiled food

Red wine

Fermented products (soy sauce, miso)

Pods of broad beans

Fava beans

Unsafe with excessive ingestion
  Sour cream
  Yogurt
  Meat extracts
  Chopped liver
  Dry sausage
  Other alcoholic beverages

*Adapted from Haddad and Winchester.

Toxic Dose: The biogenic amine interaction and hyperserotonergic syndrome may occur with therapeutic use of MAO inhibitors in the absence of overdose. Many drugs are contraindicated for those taking MAO inhibitors (Table 11). With a single ingestion of MAO inhibitors, clinical toxicity appears with doses as low as 4 mg/kg. Single ingestions of ≥6 mg/kg are often fatal. All children suspected of ingesting >4 mg/kg should be admitted to the hospital for 24 hours of observation because the appearance of severe intoxication and life-threatening manifestations may be delayed.

Diagnostic Testing: These agents are not routinely identified in a drug screen. There are no specific diagnostic tests to detect the ingestion of MAO inhibitors.

Signs and Symptoms: Clinical manifestations of MAO inhibitor intoxication depend on the cause of the intoxication. With MAO inhibitor-biogenic amine interactions, patients typically develop a severe headache associated with marked hypertension. Severe reactions produce hypertensive encephalopathy and seizures. Marked alterations in mental status or neurological examination may signal the occurrence of a cerebrovascular accident. With the hyperserotonergic syndrome, the abrupt onset of agitation, hyperpyrexia, hypertension, and skeletal muscle rigidity may occur. Seizures and severe metabolic acidosis may also appear. This syndrome may progress, with the appearance of marked myoglobinuria, renal failure, worsening acidosis, and severe cardiac dysrhythmias. Cardiac disturbances may be resistant to all treatment measures

With acute MAO inhibitor ingestion, the onset of serious toxicity may be delayed by as much as 24 hours. Early signs of toxicity may include temperature instability, dysarthria, and transient hypertension. There may be a period of apparent clinical improvement before severe toxicity, manifested by the appearance of hyperthermia, hypotension, metabolic acidosis, muscle rigidity, or rhabdomyolysis. Death occurs from cardiovascular collapse.

General Treatment: Because significant symptoms are possible, the need for life support measures including respiratory support should be anticipated.

Decontamination: (Refer to the treatment section p 6 for the appropriate use of these techniques.) Emesis can be used if instituted early. Gastric lavage with activated charcoal or activated charcoal alone should be considered if treatment is instituted later.

Antidote: No specific antidotes are available.

Specific Treatment: Hypertension can be treated with a short-acting antihypertensive agent (ie, esmolol or nitroprusside) since it may be transient. Hypotension can be treated with intravenous fluids and vasopressors. Cardiac dysrhythmias can be treated with standard agents, and severe hyperpyrexia and skeletal muscle rigidity can be treated with dantrolene. **(See Table 3, p 22, for specific dosing.)** Other interventions for moderate hyperpyrexia include the administration of acetaminophen and use of a cooling blanket.

Patient Monitoring: Laboratory monitoring should include an electrocardiogram, a urinalysis to monitor for rhabdomyolysis, and arterial blood gases and creatine phosphokinase. Cardiac monitoring is also recommended.

Enhanced Elimination: Enhanced elimination techniques are of no proven value.

References

Haddad L, Winchester J, eds. *Clinical Management of Poisoning and Drug Overdose.* 2nd ed. Philadelphia, PA: WB Saunders; 1990

Kaplan RF, Feinglass NG, Webster W, Mudra S. Phenelzine overdose treated with dantrolene sodium. *JAMA.* 1986;255:642-644

Linden CH, Rumack BH, Strehlke C. Monoamine oxidase inhibitor overdose. *Ann Emerg Med.* 1984;13:1137-1144

Lippman SB, Nash K. Monoamine oxidase inhibitor update - potential adverse food and drug interactions. *Drug Saf.* 1990;5:195-204

Mesmer RE. Don't mix miso with MAO inhibitors. *JAMA.* 1987;258:3515

Smookler S, Bermudez AJ. Hypertensive crisis resulting from an MAO inhibitor and an over-the-counter appetite suppressant. *Ann Emerg Med.* 1982;11:482-484

Opioids

Available Forms and Sources: Opioids are supplied as single agents or as a component of a variety of products used as analgesics, antitussives, and antidiarrheals. Dosage forms include tablets, capsules, liquids, rectal suppositories, and injectables. Agents discussed in this chapter include morphine, meperidine (Demerol), methadone, codeine, oxycodone (Percodan, Percocet, Tylox), pentazocine (Talwin, Talwin NX), propoxyphene (Darvon, Darvocet), hydrocodone (Hycodan), fentanyl (Sublimaze), and butorphanol (Stadol). Also included are the illicit agents heroin and opium. Diphenoxylate (Lomotil) is considered in a separate chapter (p 106).

Mechanism of Toxicity: Opioids react with at least three types of receptors widely distributed in the brain to produce a wide range of central nervous system-mediated changes.

Toxic Dose: Because most of these agents have a narrow therapeutic index, doses exceeding the therapeutic dose are likely to produce unwanted side effects or frank toxicity. The actual dose that produces toxic effects varies widely depending on the relative potency of the particular agent. Doses of 75 mg of meperidine, 10 mg of morphine or methadone, and 12.5 mg of diphenoxylate have produced respiratory depression in children. In patients toxic on opioids from combination products containing aspirin or acetaminophen, toxicity from these agents should be assessed.

Signs and Symptoms: Centrally mediated respiratory de- pression is the dominant symptom and most common cause of death. Other central nervous system signs and symptoms may include miosis (except for meperidine) lethargy, agitation, uncontrolled muscle movements, hallucinations, headache, nausea, vomiting, coma, and seizures. Pulmonary edema, sometimes associated with cardiac insufficiency, may occur. Cardiac effects may include either tachycardia or bradycardia, flushing, syncope, and cardiac arrest. Itching and urticaria are common. Hyperglycemia may also be present.

Diagnostic Testing: Most opioids can be identified qualitatively in urine drug screens. Blood levels are not clinically helpful.

General Treatment: Because significant symptoms are possible, the need for life support measures including respiratory support should be anticipated.

Decontamination: **(Refer to the treatment section p 6 for the appropriate use of these techniques.)** Emesis is contraindicated due to the rapid onset of central nervous system depression that may occur. Gastric lavage and activated charcoal treatment should be considered if a potentially toxic dose has been ingested. Cathartics should be given if activated charcoal is used, but both should be used with caution if bowel sounds are diminished or absent.

Antidote: Naloxone reverses the central nervous system and respiratory depression associated with opioid intoxication and should be given to all patients with significant symptoms **(see Table 2, p 16, for specific dosing)**. Repeated doses or a continuous infusion may be required in symptomatic patients. Larger than usual doses may be required to reverse the effects of propoxyphene.

Specific Treatment: Treatment is supportive. There is no specific treatment.

Patient Monitoring: Serum glucose levels and blood gases should be monitored in symptomatic patients.

Enhanced Elimination: Enhanced elimination techniques are of no proven value.

References

Lovejoy FH Jr, Mitchell AA, Goldman P. The management of propoxyphene poisoning. *J Pediatr.* 1974;85:98-100

Smialek JE, Monforte JR, Aronow R, Spitz WU. Methadone deaths in children: a continuing problem. *JAMA.* 1977;238:2516-2517

Phenytoin

Available Forms and Sources: Phenytoin (Dilantin) is a hydantoin compound available for oral use as chewable tablets, capsules, and a suspension. A capsule formulation in combination with phenobarbital is also marketed. New products under investigation use a prodrug, phosphenytoin, that degrades to phenytoin in vivo.

Mechanism of Toxicity: Phenytoin increases sodium-potassium ATPase pump activity and stabilizes membranes. It is also known to be directly toxic to the Purkinje cells in the cerebellum, which is the primary site of toxicity. In general, phenytoin has antidysrhythmic properties but does not cause cardio-toxic reactions. Rapid intravenous injection of phenytoin, however, can cause myocardial depression and dysrhythmias because of the vehicle it is diluted in.

Toxic Dose: Acute ingestions may cause toxicity if extremely large amounts are ingested. In general, a therapeutic loading dose of 20 mg/kg is well tolerated and thus, ingestions greater than this may be considered potentially toxic. Most phenytoin toxicity results from accumulation of the drug due to inappropriate dosing or drug-drug interactions.

Signs and Symptoms: Phenytoin does not produce the dose-related respiratory and central nervous system depression seen with many other common anticonvulsant drugs. With low but toxic concentrations (>20 μg/mL), cerebellar findings are predominant with vomiting and ataxia. Seizure activity has been reported with high concentrations, although this is not well documented. In general, coma only occurs with extremely high blood levels of phenytoin. Phenytoin inhibits the release of insulin, and severe hyperglycemia may occur.

Diagnostic Testing: Phenytoin is detected on routine drug screens. Most laboratories are able to measure levels of serum phenytoin.

General Treatment: Significant symptoms are not anticipated.

Decontamination: (Refer to the treatment section p 6 for the appropriate use of these techniques.) Emesis may be used if instituted early. Gastric lavage with activated charcoal or activated charcoal alone should be considered if treatment is delayed.

Antidote: No specific antidotes are available.

Specific Treatment: Treatment is supportive. There is no specific treatment.

Patient Monitoring: Serum glucose levels should be monitored in symptomatic patients.

Enhanced Elimination: Multiple doses of charcoal may enhance the elimination of this drug. Charcoal hemoperfusion may theoretically rapidly remove phenytoin from the circulation, although it is rarely necessary.

References

Klein JP. Diphenylhydantoin intoxication associated with hyperglycemia. *J Pediatr.* 1966;69:463-465

Larsen JR, Larsen LS. Clinical features and management of poisoning due to phenytoin. *Med Toxicol Adverse Drug Exp.* 1989;4:229-245

Masur H, Fahrendorf G, Oberwittler C, Reuther G. Cerebellar atrophy following acute intoxication with phenytoin. *Neurology.* 1990;40:1800-1801

Ros SP, Black LE. III: Multiple-dose activated charcoal in management of phenytoin overdose. *Pediatr Emerg Care.* 1989;5:169-170

Wyte CD, Berk WA. Severe oral phenytoin overdose does not cause cardiovascular morbidity. *Ann Emerg Med.* 1991;20:508-512

Quinine and Quinidine

Available Forms and Sources: Quinine sulfate, an antimalarial, is also commonly used to treat nocturnal leg cramps. It is available as tablets and capsules both over-the-counter and by prescription. Quinidine sulfate, an antidysrhythmic drug, is available in tablet, capsule, and sustained-release formulations.

Mechanism of Toxicity: These drugs are optical isomers but have slightly different toxicologic profiles. Both drugs suppress the early depolarization of the heart and are classified as Class Ia antidysrhythmics, although quinidine is more potent. Quinine causes blindness by an effect on optical nerve conduction. Both drugs have anticholinergic and α-adrenergic blocking properties.

Toxic Dose: The toxic dose of these agents is not well established. The ingestion of 5 g of quinidine was lethal in a 2-year-old; a 16-year-old survived an overdose of 8 g. Quinine ingestions greater than 4 g must be considered potentially lethal.

Signs and Symptoms: Both drugs cause central nervous system depression, although respiratory depression is not a prominent effect.

Quinidine toxicity. Headache, tinnitus, and choreoathetosis, nausea, vomiting, diarrhea, and generalized weakness have been described. Cardiac effects include tachycardia, hypertension or hypotension, atrioventricular block, intraventricular block, ventricular dysrhythmia, prolongation of the QTc and QRS duration, and asystole.

Quinine toxicity. Nervous system symptoms include headache, tinnitus, choreoathetosis, deafness, mutism, seizures, and generalized weakness. Nausea, vomiting, and diarrhea may also be seen. Fixed and dilated pupils, blurred vision, halos, reduced corneal sensitivity, constriction of the visual fields, total blindness, narrowing of the retinal arteries, and retinal edema can develop. Central visual acuity usually returns to normal but fields may be permanently constricted. Cardiac signs include tachycardia, hypertension or hypotension, atrioventricular block, intraventricular block, ventricular dysrhythmia, and prolongation of QTc and QRS intervals. Disseminated intravascular coagulation on a immunologic basis has been reported in adults.

Diagnostic Testing: These agents are usually detected in a routine drug screen. Serum levels of both drugs are commonly available. Some assays measure metabolites as well as the parent compound. Toxic levels are ill defined; toxicity, however, is likely to occur at levels >8 mg/L for either drug.

General Treatment: Following significant exposure, all patients should undergo continuous cardiac monitoring for at least 6 hours.

Decontamination: (Refer to the treatment section p 6 for the appropriate use of these techniques.) Emesis, gastric lavage, or activated charcoal therapy should be considered if a potentially toxic dose has been ingested and treatment is instituted early. Gastric lavage with activated charcoal or activated charcoal alone may also be used.

Antidote: No specific antidotes are available.

Specific Treatment: (See Table 3, p 22, for specific dosing.) Isoproterenol can be administered to treat bradycardia. Norepinephrine can be used to treat hypotension. Ventricular dysrhythmias should be treated with boluses of sodium bicarbonate repeated frequently enough to maintain a blood pH of approximately 7.5. Treat seizures with benzodiazepines as required.

Patient Monitoring: A baseline complete blood count and an electrocardiogram should be obtained and monitored.

Enhanced Elimination: Multiple doses of activated charcoal may increase elimination. Forced diuresis also increases the urinary elimination of these drugs; the fluid overload required for this therapy, however, may be dangerous if the cardiac output is compromised.

References

Baselt RC, Cravey RH. *Disposition of Toxic Drugs and Chemicals in Man.* 3rd ed. Chicago, IL: Year Book Medical Publishers; 1989:743-750

Dellocchio T, Pailli F, Testa O, Vergassola R. Accidental quinidine poisoning in two children. *Pediatrics.* 1976;58:288-290

Dyson EH, Proudfoot AT, Bateman DN. Quinine amblyopia: is current management appropriate? *Clin Toxicol.* 1985-1986;23:571-578

Garrettson LK, Geller RJ. Acid and alkaline diuresis: when are they of value in the treatment of poisoning. *Drug Saf.* 1990;5:220-232

Grattan-Smith TM, Gillis J, Kilham H. Quinine poisoning in children. *Med J Aust.* 1987;147:93-95

Kim SY, Benowitz NL. Poisoning due to class Ia antiarrhythmic drugs: quinidine, procainamide, and disopyramide. *Drug Saf.* 1990;5:393-420

Prescott LF, Hamilton AR, Heyworth R. Treatment of quinine overdosage with repeated oral charcoal. *Br J Clin Pharmacol.* 1989;27:95-97

Schonwald S, Shannon M. Unsuspected quinine intoxication presenting as acute deafness and mutism. *Am J Emerg Med.* 1991;9:318-320

Thomas D. Forced acid diuresis and stellate ganglion block in the treatment of quinine poisoning. *Anesthesia.* 1984;39:257-260

Salicylates

Available Forms and Sources: Aspirin (acetylsalicylic acid) is supplied as tablets, chewable tablets, and rectal suppositories and is also available as an effervescent tablet or in chewing gum form. Sodium salicylate is supplied as tablets. Both products also come as enteric–coated tablets and are found in cold and analgesic mixtures as tablets, capsules, powder, or liquids.

Methyl salicylate is available as oil of wintergreen and as an ingredient in analgesic ointments and liniments. Other sources of salicylates include magnesium salicylate and choline salicylate (Trilisate), choline salicylate (Arthropan), magnesium salicylate (Doan's Pills), and bismuth subsalicylate (Peptobismol).

Mechanism of Toxicity: Salicylates directly stimulate the respiratory center in the brain, uncouple oxidative phosphorylation, inhibit Krebs cycle enzymes, and inhibit amino acid metabolism, thereby interfering with homeostatic mechanisms.

In addition, aspirin is a gastric irritant, decreases platelet adhesiveness, and inhibits the synthesis of clotting factor VII, creating some risk of bleeding.

Toxic Dose: The acute toxic dose of aspirin is 150 mg/kg. One milliliter of oil of wintergreen (99% methyl salicylate) is equivalent to 1.4 g of aspirin in salicylate potency.

Signs and Symptoms: Nausea and vomiting are common. As a result of direct respiratory stimulation, hyperpnea and hyperventilation are prominent, resulting in respiratory alkalosis. In adults and adolescents, alkalosis may persist until terminal respiratory failure develops. In young children, respiratory alkalosis is combined with metabolic acidosis because of the accumulation of lactic acid and other organic acids. When patients of all ages are considered, respiratory alkalosis with metabolic acidosis is most common (50%), followed by respiratory alkalosis alone (20%) and metabolic acidosis alone (20%), followed by combined respiratory and metabolic acidosis (10%). Dehydration and electrolyte imbalance generally occur with oliguria secondary to inadequate renal perfusion or excess antidiuretic hormone secretion. Fever and sweating contribute to dehydration. Electrolyte derangements include hyperkalemia, hypokalemia, hypernatremia, or hyponatremia. Central nervous system symptoms include headache, tinnitus, irritability, restlessness, delirium, hallucinations, confusion, mania, convulsions, or coma.

Transient hyperglycemia and glycosuria are common; small children may develop hypoglycemia. Other complications include hemorrhagic diathesis from inhibition of prothrombin synthesis or platelet dysfunction and cerebral or pulmonary edema. Death results from respiratory failure, cardiovascular collapse, electrolyte imbalance, or cerebral edema.

Diagnostic Testing: Salicylates are detected on a routine drug screen or may be identified qualitatively by a positive ferric chloride test on blood or urine. Salicylates are readily quantified in blood and levels should be obtained at least 6 hours following ingestion to allow for interpretation on the nomogram (Fig 3). Levels <35 mg/dL at 6 hours are associated with no symptoms, 35 to 70 mg/dL with mild symptoms, and 70 to 100 mg/dL with severe symptoms. Levels >150 mg/dL are potentially fatal (see Fig 3). At a given salicylate level, chronic poisoning exhibits much more severe clinical findings than acute poisoning. The nomogram cannot be used to interpret salicylate levels after a chronic exposure.

General Treatment: Significant acute symptoms are not anticipated.

Decontamination: (Refer to the treatment section p 6 for the appropriate use of these techniques). Emesis, gastric lavage, or activated charcoal should be considered if a potentially toxic dose

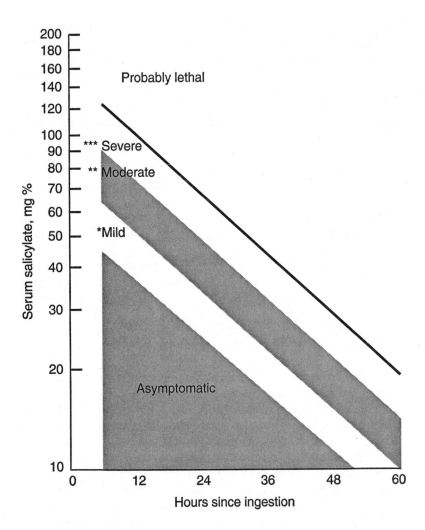

Fig 3. Nonogram relating serum salicylate level to severity of intoxication at varying intervals after acute ingestion of single doses of aspirin. Nomogram starts at 6 hours to ensure that levels will not be interpreted before they have reached their peak; it can be used earlier if more than one level is obtained to establish that the salicylate level is declining. *Mild toxicity: Mild to moderate hyperpnea without acidosis, lethargy, and vomiting. Slight fever may be present. **Moderate toxicity: Severe hyperpnea with acidosis, marked lethargy or excitability but no coma or convulsions, and marked gastrointestinal distress. ***Severe toxicity: Severe hyperpnea, severe neurologic impairment that may include coma or convulsions, and marked metabolic acidosis. Adapted from Done AK: Aspirin overdose: incidence, diagnosis and management. *Pediatrics.* 1978;62(suppl):895.

has been ingested. Significant amounts of salicylate may be present in the gastrointestinal tract of patients who ingest large amounts even as long as 12 hours after ingestion.

Antidote: No specific antidotes are available.

Specific Treatment: Fluids, electrolytes, and glucose should be administered as required to correct dehydration, acidosis, hypoglycemia, and electrolyte imbalance. If the patient is in shock, plasma or albumin (10 to 15 mL/kg) should be administered. A good urine flow should be established. Sodium bicarbonate may be given for acidosis until the blood pH is normalized, thereby preventing distribution of salicylate into tissues. In children older than 4 years, the serum bicarbonate concentration may be decreased, but the pH of the blood is generally normal or high (alkalotic). This alkalosis is caused by direct stimulation of the respiratory center by salicylates with respiratory alkalosis predominating over a metabolic acidosis. In this situation, bicarbonate must be administered more cautiously. The aim of bicarbonate therapy is to maintain the blood pH within the normal range and the urine pH above 7.5. Alkalinization of the urine greatly increases the clearance of salicylates. When urine output is adequate, potassium chloride should be added to the intravenous fluids at a concentration of 3.0 to 4.0 mEq/L in order to prevent paradoxical aciduria. The usual fluid requirement during the period of severe symptoms is 2.5 to 4.0 L/M^2/d. With severe acidosis, large amounts of sodium bicarbonate may be required to correct the acid base balance. Tetany should be treated by cessation of bicarbonate therapy and intravenous administration of calcium gluconate. Respiratory depression may require artificial ventilation and oxygen. Seizures can be controlled with diazepam or barbiturates, and hyperpyrexia should be treated with external cooling. Vitamin K should be given parenterally to correct hypoprothrombinemia.

Patient Monitoring: Obtain blood samples for determination of the following values: salicylate, pH, pCO$_2$, bicarbonate, sodium, potassium, chloride, and glucose. The frequency of monitoring is determined by the clinical course. The Done nomogram (Fig 3) may assist in evaluating the severity of intoxication if the salicylate was ingested in a single dose.

Enhanced Elimination: The use of hemodialysis may be indicated in patients with salicylate levels >100 to 120 mg/dL when salicylate cannot be removed because of renal or hepatic failure, or when response to conservative therapy is inadequate. Dialysis may be needed at much lower serum levels of salicylate following chronic poisoning.

References

Brenner BE, Simon RR. Management of salicylate intoxication. Drugs. 1982;24:335-340

Curtis RA, Barone J, Giacona N. Efficacy of ipecac and activated charcoal/cathartic: prevention of salicylate absorption in a simulated overdose. *Arch Intern Med.* 1984;144:48-52

Gaudreault P, Temple AR, Lovejoy FH Jr. The relative severity of acute versus chronic salicylate poisoning in children: a clinical comparison. *Pediatrics.* 1982;70:566-569

McGuigan MA. A two-year review of salicylate deaths in Ontario. *Arch Intern Med.* 1987;147:510-512

Temple AR. Acute and chronic effects of aspirin toxicity and their treatment. *Arch Intern Med.* 1981;141:364-369

Sedative Hypnotic Agents

Available Forms and Sources: The sedative hypnotic agents discussed in this section include ethchlorvynol (Placidyl), glutethimide (Doriden), meprobamate (Equanil, Miltown), methyprylon (Noludar), and zolpidem (Ambien). These drugs are available as tablets or capsules. In addition, see the sections on barbiturates (p 52), benzodiazepines (p 55), chloral hydrate (p 69), and methaqualone (p 160).

Mechanism of Toxicity: The specific mechanisms vary among substances but in general are due to direct central nervous system depression.

Toxic Dose: The toxic dose is variable and is not well defined in the literature.

Signs and Symptoms: A decrease in the level of consciousness ranging from lethargy to coma is seen in all significant sedative hypnotic overdoses. Ingestion of most of these drugs can also produce cardiorespiratory depression and arrest.

Diagnostic Testing: These agents are not routinely identified in a drug screen. Specific serum drug concentrations are of no clinical value.

General Treatment: Because significant symptoms are possible, the need for life support measures including cardiorespiratory support should be anticipated.

Decontamination: (Refer to the treatment section p 6 for the appropriate use of these techniques.) Emesis should be avoided due to the possibility of central nervous system depression. Gastric lavage with activated charcoal or activated charcoal treatment alone should be considered if a potentially toxic dose has been ingested.

Antidote: No specific antidotes are available.

Specific Treatment: Treatment is supportive. There is no specific treatment.

Patient Monitoring: Monitor the patient's level of consciousness and cardiac rate and rhythm.

Enhanced Elimination: The use of hemodialysis or hemoperfusion has been reported with some of these agents; there are little objective data, however, that it improves outcome and should probably be reserved for only the most severe cases. Repeated doses of activated charcoal may increase the elimination of active glutethimide metabolites that undergo enterohepatic recirculation.

References

Bertino JS Jr, Reed MD. Barbiturate and nonbarbiturate sedative hypnotic intoxication in children. *Pediatr Clin North Am.* 1986;33:703

Dennison J, Edwards N, Volans GN. Meprobamate overdosage. *Vet Hum Toxicol*. 1985;4:215-217

Gomolin I. Ethchlorvynol. *Clin Toxicol Rev*. 1980;2:1-2

Steroids

Available Forms and Sources: A wide variety of agents with glucocorticoid, mineralocorticoid, and androgenic properties are marketed. Common agents include hydrocortisone, prednisone, dexamethasone, methylprednisolone, and fludrocortisone, which are available in oral, injectable, and topical dosage forms.

Mechanism of Toxicity: Toxicity results from an extension of therapeutic effects.

Toxic Dose: Acute ingestion rarely results in systemic toxic reactions. Toxicity would only be expected from chronic ingestion over a minimum of several weeks.

Signs and Symptoms: Acute gastrointestinal upset manifested by abdominal pain and vomiting can be a consequence of large ingestions.

Diagnostic Testing: These agents are not detected in a routine drug screen. Blood level monitoring is not clinically useful.

General Treatment: Care is usually unnecessary due to the low inherent toxicity of these products.

Decontamination: Gastrointestinal decontamination is usually not necessary and therefore is not recommended.

Antidote: No specific antidotes are available.

Specific Treatment: Treatment is supportive. There is no specific treatment.

Patient Monitoring: No specific monitoring is necessary.

Enhanced Elimination: Enhanced elimination techniques are of
no proven value.

References

Eberlein WR, Bongiovanni AM, Rodriguez CS. Diagnosis and treatment:
the complications of steroid treatment. *Pediatrics.* 1967;40:279-282

Feiwel M, James VH, Barnett ES. Effect of potent topical steroids on
plasma-cortisol levels of infants and children with eczema. *Lancet.*
1969;1:485-487

Hollman GA, Allen DB. Overt glucocorticoid excess due to inhaled corti-
costeroid treatment. *Pediatrics.* 1988;81:452-455

Sympathomimetics

Available Forms and Sources: Sympathomimetics are
widely used as decongestants and as weight-reduction aids. Compounds included in this category are ephedrine, pseudoephedrine,
phenylephrine, and phenylpropanolamine. They are available
alone or in combination with antihistamines and analgesics
in prescription and over-the-counter formulations and are frequently an ingredient in "street speed" preparations.

Mechanism of Toxicity: Sympathomimetics act either directly
by stimulating adrenergic receptors, or indirectly by stimulating
the release of endogenous catecholamines that stimulate adrenergic receptors. Nonamphetamine sympathomimetics have low
potency and little penetration into the central nervous system.
They have low abuse potential when compared to amphetamines.

Toxic Dose: Toxic doses are not well defined in the literature.
Doses above five times the usual total daily dose may produce
significant symptoms.

Signs and Symptoms: After severe sympathomimetic ingestions, clinical manifestations can include agitation, hyperpyrexia,
hypertension, tachycardia, and seizures. Rarely, cardiac dysrhythmias may occur. Phenylpropanolamine is a selective α-adrenergic
agonist that causes profound hypertension without tachycardia;

this may be associated with hypertensive encephalopathy, including seizures, or cerebrovascular hemorrhage.

Diagnostic Testing: Most sympathomimetics are readily detected as amphetamines in urine by immunoassay. Depending on the specific agent and urine pH, the drug may be detected in urine 20 to 30 hours after ingestion. Quantitative measures in blood are not clinically useful.

General Treatment: Significant symptoms are not expected unless large amounts have been ingested.

Decontamination: (Refer to the treatment section p 6 for the appropriate use of these techniques.) Emesis should be considered if a potentially toxic dose has been ingested and treatment is instituted early. Gastric lavage with activated charcoal or activated charcoal treatment alone may also be used.

Antidote: No specific antidotes are available.

Specific Treatment: (See Table 3, p 22, for specific dosing.) Seizures may be treated with benzodiazepines. Hypertensive crises, particularly those that occur after phenylpropanolamine intoxication, should be treated immediately with a short-acting antihypertensive agent such as nitroprusside or nifedipine. Agitation can generally be controlled with haloperidol or a benzodiazepine.

Patient Monitoring: Obtain a urinalysis and determinations for levels of creatine phosphokinase and arterial blood gases and monitor the electrocardiogram in symptomatic patients. Computed tomography should be performed if the patient has an unexplained altered mental status.

Enhanced Elimination: Forced acid diuresis theoretically can increase the elimination of sympathomimetics; urine acidification, however, typically requires administration of ammonium chloride, which creates a metabolic acidosis. Because of the concurrent risk of myoglobinuria and the systemic effects of metabolic acidosis, urine acidification is not recommended after sympathomimetic overdose. Hemodialysis is also an effective means of enhancing elimination of sympathomimetics but is rarely necessary and should be reserved for cases with renal failure.

References

Forman HP, Levin S, Stewart B, Patel M, Feinstein S. Cerebral vasculitis and hemorrhage in an adolescent taking diet pills containing phenylpropanolamine: case report and review of literature. *Pediatrics.* 1989; 83:737-741

Gibson RG, Oliver JA, Leak D. Nifedipine therapy of phenylpropanolamine-induced hypertension. *Am Heart J.* 1987;113:406-407

Pentel P. Toxicity of over-the-counter stimulants. *JAMA.* 1984;252:1898-1903

Sawyer DR, Conner CS, Rumack BH. Managing acute toxicity for nonprescription stimulants. *Clin Pharm.* 1982;1:529-533

Theophylline

Available Forms and Sources: Theophylline is a methylxanthine alkaloid available in liquid, capsule, tablet, and sustained-release formulations. Aminophylline is the ethylenediamine salt of theophylline and is available orally and parenterally. Aminophylline is about 80% theophylline. Table 13 contains the percentage of anhydrous theophylline in various salts.

Table 13. Percentage of Anhydrous Theophylline

Preparation	Percentage of Anhydrous Theophylline
Aminophylline anhydrous	85
Aminophylline hydrous	79
Dyphyllin	0
Theophylline	
Calcium salicylate	50
Monohydrate	90
Sodium glycinate	48

Mechanism of Toxicity: Although phosphodiesterase inhibition of the breakdown of cyclic adenosine monophosphate was once thought to be the primary mechanism of theophylline effects, it is now unclear. Several mechanisms have been proposed—inhibition of prostaglandin action, stimulation of catecholamine action, adenosine receptor antagonism, translocation of intracellular calcium, and other factors, including enhanced contraction of the muscles of the diaphragm.

Aminophylline can cause allergic reactions that may initially be seen as delayed hypersensitivity 12 to 24 hours after exposure.

Toxic Dose: Acute toxicity is affected by the type of preparation ingested, route of exposure, age-related clearance rate, physical condition of the patient, and drug and nondrug interactions. Single doses greater than 10 mg/kg can produce mild toxicity. Doses over 20 mg/kg may produce moderate toxicity. As a general rule, a single dose of 1 mg/kg produces a serum theophylline concentration (STC) of approximately 2 µg/mL. An estimate of STC can be obtained by the following equation:

$$STC \ (\mu g/mL) = \frac{\text{dose of theophylline in mg}}{\text{wt (kg)} \times V_d}$$

$$V_d = 0.45 L/kg$$

The correlation of blood concentrations with acute toxicity is described in Table 14. The toxic effects following chronic theophylline overdose do not correlate with plasma drug concentrations.

Signs and Symptoms: Theophylline overdose affects the gastrointestinal tract, central nervous system, and cardiovascular system. Gastrointestinal symptoms in mild toxicity include anorexia, nausea, and vomiting. More severe intoxications produce hematemesis or coffee ground vomitus. Sustained-release preparations produce mild or no gastrointestinal symptoms.

Cardiovascular effects in mild toxicity include sinus tachycardia and premature ventricular contractions. Moderate intoxication is associated with hypertension due to cardiac stimulation or hypotension due to a decrease in peripheral vascular resistance. Severe intoxication can produce supraventricular tachycardia

Table 14. Correlation of Blood Theophylline Concentrations With Acute Toxicity*

Plasma Concentration, µg/mL	Toxicity Degree	Manifestations
8 - 10	None	Bronchodilation
10 - 20	Mild	Therapeutic range, nausea, vomiting, insomnia, nervousness and irritability, tachycardia, respiratory alkalosis
20 - 40	Moderate	Gastrointestinal complaints and central nervous system stimulation, agitation, restlessness, tremor, headache, abdominal pain, convulsions, transient hypertension, hyperthermia, tachypnea
>60	Severe	Convulsions and dysrhythmias (may occur at lower levels and without gastrointestinal symptoms). Children tolerate higher serum concentrations. Sinus tachycardia, electrolyte abnormalities, hyperglycemia
>100	Very severe	Tachydysrhythmias, seizures, acid-base abnormalities

*The data in this table do not apply to cases involving chronic toxicity.

(SVT) and ventricular dysrhythmias, but sustained dysrhythmias that require prolonged therapy are rare. The most common dysrhythmia is SVT.

Central nervous system effects include agitation, tremulousness, headache, confusion, and insomnia. In acute intoxication seizures are infrequent and are usually focal and brief. Seizures are usually preceded by other effects but may occur without warning. The onset of seizures may be delayed for as long as 10 to 12 hours after the ingestion of sustained-release preparations. In chronic intoxications seizures may be the presenting sign and are protracted and difficult to control. Hallucinations have been reported.

Rhabdomyolysis may occur, causing myoglobinuria, renal failure, and acute compartment syndrome. Hypokalemia occurs early and correlates with blood levels. Hypokalemia may contribute to cardiac dysrhythmias and is the result of potassium movement into cells, loss of potassium with vomiting, and the diuretic action of theophylline. Hyperglycemia due to catecholamine release and glycogenolysis may occur. Hypercalcemia, hypophosphatemia, and elevation in levels of amylase and uric acid have been noted. Leukocytosis, severe metabolic lactic acidosis, and dehydration may develop in severe intoxications.

Chronic intoxication is often more serious and difficult to treat. Following chronic exposures the blood level does not correlate with toxicity the way it does following acute exposures. An STC of 90 to 110 µg/mL may be seen in acutely intoxicated patients without morbidity and mortality but concentrations >60 µg/mL in chronic intoxications are associated with increased mortality. Electrolyte abnormalities are not features of chronic intoxication. Dysrhythmias may occur when STCs are >30 to 40 µg/mL with seizures at >40 µg/mL in chronic intoxications. Therapeutic intervention is recommended at much lower STCs (>60 µg/mL) in chronic intoxication regardless of the patient's symptoms.

Diagnostic Testing: Theophylline is detected in most routine drug screens and quantitation can be done in most laboratories. Because it is the unbound drug that exerts its pharmacologic effect and the concentration of bound and unbound theophylline is commonly measured by hospital laboratories, patients with low albumin levels may have manifestations of toxicity despite a normal blood level of the drug. It is advisable to check the serum albumin levels in such patients.

Peak STCs occur within 1 hour after the ingestion of liquid preparations, 1 to 3 hours after regular release preparations, and 3 to 24 hours after slow-release preparations.

General Treatment: Because significant symptoms are possible, the need for life support measures including respiratory support and treatment of seizures should be anticipated.

Decontamination: (Refer to the treatment section p 6 for the appropriate use of these techniques.) In severe overdose, use gastric lavage, activated charcoal treatment, or both, up to 4 hours after ingestion with regular preparations and up to 8 to 12 hours with slow-release preparations. Emesis is not recommended because of the rapid onset of seizures. Activated charcoal is extremely effective in reducing STCs. Whole bowel irrigation may be useful when sustained-release preparations have been ingested. Endoscopic removal of concretions may be necessary in extreme cases.

Antidote: No specific antidotes are available.

Specific Treatment: (See Table 3, p 22, for specific dosing.) Seizures can be controlled with diazepam or phenobarbital. Phenytoin is often ineffective in controlling seizures. Seizures following chronic intoxication are often refractory and may require paralyzing agents and assisted ventilation.

Dysrhythmias can be treated with appropriate agents. Propranolol and nonselective β-blockers should not be used to control SVT in asthmatic patients because they may produce bronchospasm. Even cardiospecific β-blockers may cause bronchospasm in asthmatic patients and these agents are reserved for life-threatening SVT. Esmolol, a cardioselective short-acting β-blocker, has been successful in controlling dysrhythmias and is being investigated. Lidocaine, which is the treatment of choice for ventricular dysrhythmias, may potentially cause seizures. Verapamil has been successfully used to treat multifocal atrial tachycardia; increased mortality has been reported when verapamil therapy is used, however, and therefore it is not recommended. Adenosine treatment is ineffective. Avoid drugs that increase the QT interval such as quinidine and disopyramide, until hypokalemia is corrected. Mexiletine therapy is associated with decreased theophylline elimination and should be avoided.

Hypotension can be treated with positioning and fluids and, if necessary, vasopressors, with a preference for norepinephrine as opposed to dopamine therapy. Hypertension rarely requires therapy, but if emergency therapy is needed, nitroprusside is recommended. Hyperglycemia is usually mild and does not require insulin therapy.

Massive hematemesis can be managed with saline lavage and blood replacement, if needed. Antacids may be given, but histamine$_2$ blockers such as cimetidine interfere with theophylline metabolism and should be avoided. If intractable vomiting occurs, an antiemetic such as metoclopramide or droperidol can be administered.

Patient Monitoring: Determine if occult blood is present in vomitus and stools and monitor the hemoglobin level and hematocrit value. Monitor the patient's electrocardiogram, renal and hepatic function, acid-base balance, and levels of electrolytes, calcium, blood glucose, serum creatine kinase, urine myoglobin, and arterial blood gases. Obtain theophylline blood concentrations serially every 4 hours (especially with overdoses of slow-release preparations) until a plateau is reached, then monitor the concentrations every 6 to 8 hours until levels are below 20 µg/mL. Increases in STCs despite decontamination may indicate concretions or the ingestion of a slow-release preparation.

Enhanced Elimination: Hemodialysis is of little benefit unless renal failure occurs. Repeated doses of activated charcoal are effective in acute and chronic ingestions as well as intravenous overdoses. Whole bowel irrigation may assist in removing retained sustained-release preparations.

Charcoal hemoperfusion enhances the elimination of theophylline and can prevent seizures and dysrhythmias. The indications for charcoal hemoperfusion include patients aged 6 months to 60 years with STCs >80 to 100 µg/mL in acute intoxications and >40 to 60 µg/mL in chronic intoxications; the presence of intractable uncontrollable seizures or dysrhythmias regardless of the STC; the inability to tolerate activated charcoal despite antiemetic therapy with persistent elevation in STC after 6 to 8 hours; and extensive hematemesis with persistent elevation of the STC.

References

American Academy of Pediatrics, Committee on Drugs. Precautions concerning the use of theophylline. *Pediatrics.* 1992;89:781-783

Anderson W, Youl B, Mackay IR. Acute theophylline intoxication. *Ann Emerg Med.* 1991;20:1143-1145

Baker MD. Theophylline toxicity in children. *J Pediatr.* 1986;109:538-542

Bernard S. Severe lactic acidosis following theophylline overdose. *Ann Emerg Med.* 1991;20:1135-1137

Hendeles L, Weinberger M, Szefler S, Ellis E. Safety and efficacy of theophylline in children with asthma. *J Pediatr.* 1992;120:177-183

Olson KR, Benowitz NL, Woo OF, Pond SM. Theophylline overdose: acute single ingestion vs chronic repeated overmedication. *Am J Emerg Med.* 1985;3:386-394

Powell EC, Reynolds SL, Rubenstein JS. Theophylline toxicity in children: a retrospective review. *Pediatr Emerg Care.* 1993;9:129-133

Schlieper A, Alcock D, Beaudry P, Feldman W, Leikin L. Effect of therapeutic plasma concentrations of theophylline on behavior, cognitive processing, and effect in children with asthma. *J Pediatr.* 1991;118:449-455

Sessler CN. Theophylline toxicity: clinical features of 116 cases. *Am J Med.* 1990;88:567-576

Shannon M, Amitai Y, Lovejoy FH Jr. Multiple-dose activated charcoal for theophylline poisoning in young infants. *Pediatrics.* 1987;80:368-370

Shannon M, Lovejoy FH Jr. Effect of acute versus chronic intoxication on the clinical features of theophylline poisoning in children. *J Pediatr.* 1992;121:125-130

Skinner MH. Adverse reactions and interactions with theophylline. *Drug Saf.* 1990;5:275-285

Thyroid Hormones

Available Forms and Sources: Thyroid hormone products include thyroid (USP), containing natural or desiccated thyroid (triiodothyronine [T_3] and thyroxine [T_4]); liothyronine (synthetic T_3, Cytomel); levothyroxine (synthetic T_4, Synthroid); and synthetic T_4 and T_3 in a ratio of 4:1 (liotrix).

Mechanism of Toxicity: Thyroid hormones stimulate the cardiovascular, gastrointestinal, and cardiovascular systems.

Toxic Dose: The toxic dose is not well defined; symptoms may be expected following ingestions of greater than 3 mg of levothyroxine, 6 grains of desiccated thyroid, or 0.75 mg of liothyronine.

Signs and Symptoms: The onset of symptoms following acute ingestion of T_3-containing products may be delayed 4 to 12 hours. Clinical effects include nausea, vomiting, diarrhea, fever, hyperactive behavior, diaphoresis, flushing, irritability, lethargy, abdominal pain, and supraventricular tachycardia. Clinical effects following ingestions of levothyroxine are similar but may be delayed for 5 to 7 days.

Diagnostic Testing: T_3 and T_4 are not detected in a routine drug screen. Serum levels of T_3 and T_4 may be monitored but are not prognostic and do not correlate well with symptoms. Levels should be obtained at least 6 hours after exposure. Significant elevations in levels may identify patients requiring follow-up 5 to 7 days after ingestion.

General Treatment: Significant acute symptoms are not anticipated.

Decontamination: (Refer to the treatment section p 6 for the appropriate use of these techniques.) Emesis can be used if instituted early. Gastric lavage with activated charcoal or activated charcoal treatment alone may also be used.

Antidote: No antidotes are available.

Specific Treatment: (See Table 3, p 22, for specific dosing.) Propranolol may be used to treat adrenergic symptoms. Propylthiouracil inhibits the conversion of T_4 to T_3; its clinical usefulness in acute overdose, however, is unclear. Sodium ipodate inhibits the peripheral conversion of T_4 to T_3. The dose is 3.1 g/1.7 m². Its clinical usefulness in acute overdose is unclear. Acetaminophen can be used for symptomatic treatment of fever.

Patient Monitoring: Patients should be monitored for cardiac disturbances and fluid and electrolyte imbalance.

Enhanced Elimination: Forced diuresis and hemodialysis are not effective. Exchange transfusion has been used with limited success in severe cases. Charcoal hemoperfusion may be of value for massive ingestions.

References

Litovitz TL, White JD. Levothyroxine ingestions in children: analysis of 78 cases. *Am J Emerg Med.* 1985;3:209-300

Lewander WJ, Lacouture PG, Silva JE, Lovejoy FH. Acute thyroxine ingestion in pediatric patients. *Pediatrics.* 1989;84:262-265

Valproic Acid

Available Forms and Sources: Valproic acid is formulated as tablets, capsules, sprinkle capsules, and a suspension. Depakene is a brand name for valproic acid, and Depakote is a brand name for divalproex sodium, which is a mixture of valproic acid and sodium valproate and is a sustained-release formulation. The strength is expressed in terms of the amount of valproic acid.

Mechanism of Toxicity: Valproic acid increases the effects of gamma-aminobutyric acid (GABA) in the central nervous system. Valproic acid is also hepatotoxic, although the mechanism is unclear.

Toxic Dose: Toxic effects may develop following an ingestion of more than the usual daily dose of 15 to 25 mg/kg. More commonly, toxicity is associated with long-term therapy at excessive doses or when drug interactions occur resulting in toxic serum concentrations.

Signs and Symptoms: Central nervous system effects may be seen with depressed levels of consciousness and, rarely, seizure activity and coma. Asterixis and hallucinations have been reported. Hepatotoxicity (described as a Reyes syndrome-like effect) is not generally associated with acute intoxication. A single case report of pancreatitis and bone marrow depression associated with a single large ingestion has been reported.

Diagnostic Testing: Valproic acid is not detected by most routine drug screens. Valproate levels, however, are widely available. Serum concentrations in excess of 150 µg/mL are considered to be toxic. Occasionally therapeutic concentrations closer to 200 µg/mL have been used without toxicity.

General Treatment: Significant symptoms are not anticipated.

Decontamination: (Refer to the treatment section p 6 for the appropriate use of these techniques.) Emesis can be used if instituted early. Gastric lavage with activated charcoal or activated charcoal treatment alone may also be used.

Antidote: No specific antidotes are available.

Specific Treatment: Reversal of coma with naloxone has been reported in a single case.

Patient Monitoring: Following large single doses or with long-term toxicity, evaluation of levels of ammonia and liver function studies may be appropriate. Given the case report of pancreatitis, monitoring of serum amylase levels may be appropriate under the same circumstances.

Enhanced Elimination: Although it has been demonstrated that dialysis and charcoal hemoperfusion can remove this compound, the role of these treatment modalities for the management of severe ingestion is unclear because the consequences of the ingestion are usually mild.

References

Alberto G, Erickson T, Popiel R, Narayanan M, Hryhorczuk D. Central nervous system manifestations of a valproic acid overdose responsive to naloxone. *Ann Emerg Med.* 1989;18:889-891

Garnier R, Boudignat O, Fournier PE. Valproate poisoning. *Lancet.* 1982;2:97

Janssen F, Rambeck B, Schnabel R. Acute valproate intoxication with fatal outcome in an infant. *Neuropediatrics.* 1985;16:235-238

Khoo SH, Leyland MJ. Cerebral edema following acute sodium valproate overdose. *J Toxicol Clin Toxicol.* 1992;30:209-214

Roodhooft AM, Van Dam K, Haentjens D, Verpooten GA, Van Acker KJ. Acute sodium valproate intoxication: occurrence of renal failure and treatment with haemoperfusion-haemodialysis. *Eur J Pediatr.* 1990;149:363-364

Vitamins (Excluding Iron)

Available Forms and Sources: Fat-soluble vitamins include vitamin A, vitamin E, and vitamin D. Water-soluble vitamins include ascorbic acid (vitamin C), folic acid, riboflavin (B$_2$), thiamine (B$_1$), cyanocobalamin (B$_{12}$), biotin, pantothenic acid, pyridoxine (B_6), and niacin. Minerals and trace elements include calcium, chromium, phosphorous, iodine, iron, magnesium, copper, zinc, manganese, and selenium. Products are formulated with a variety of ingredients in a variety of concentrations as tablets, chewable tablets, capsules, and liquids. Preparations containing iron are much more likely to produce toxicity (see iron management section, p 96).

Mechanism of Toxicity: The mechanism of toxicity for vitamin A is not known. Vitamin D enhances the absorption of calcium from the gastrointestinal tract with the potential for hypercalcemia. Niacin stimulates histamine release.

Toxic Dose: Multiple-vitamin preparations have a wide margin of safety and even large ingestions produce only mild symptoms. A single dose of 75 000 IU of vitamin A in infants and 12 000 IU/kg in older children may produce symptoms. Doses of niacin greater than 100 mg may produce mild symptoms. Acute toxicity following a single dose of vitamin D is unlikely. It is estimated that ingesting >25 000 IU of vitamin D per day for a month or more is necessary to develop toxicity. Toxic reactions from other constituents of vitamin preparations (except iron) are highly unlikely.

Signs and Symptoms: Large doses of multiple-vitamin preparations may produce symptoms of nausea, vomiting, and diarrhea, which are usually self-limiting. Discoloration of urine (intense yellow due to riboflavin) and feces may occur.

Vitamin A can produce nausea, vomiting, diarrhea, irritability, and bulging fontanelles with elevated cerebrospinal fluid pressure. Niacin can cause pruritus and cutaneous flushing and may aggravate asthma. Vitamin D may produce hypercalcemia following chronic ingestion.

Diagnostic Testing: These agents are not detected on a routine drug screen. In general, vitamin levels are not useful to assess acute exposures. Vitamin A levels, if available, may aid in confirming the diagnosis.

General Treatment: Significant symptoms are not anticipated even following large ingestions.

Decontamination: (Refer to the treatment section p 6 for the appropriate use of these techniques.) Gastrointestinal decontamination is usually not necessary. For ingestions of toxic quantities of vitamin A, emesis, gastric lavage, or activated charcoal therapy should be considered.

Antidote: No specific antidotes are available.

Specific Treatment: For vitamin A toxicity, intracranial pressure can be reduced with mannitol or steroid therapy. For niacin toxicity, treatment with antihistamines may relieve pruritus. Hypercalcemia secondary to vitamin D usually does not require treatment; saline diuresis, however, can be used.

Patient Monitoring: Measure the patient's intracranial pressure and serum calcium level, if indicated.

Enhanced Elimination: Enhanced elimination techniques are of no proven value.

Reference

Dean BS, Krenzelok EP. Multiple vitamins and vitamins with iron: accidental poisoning in children. *Vet Hum Toxicol*. 1988;30:23-25

ABUSE DRUGS

Amphetamines

Available Forms and Sources: All amphetamines and amphetamine-like compounds are controlled substances and legally available only by prescription. Agents included are amphetamine, dextroamphetamine (Dexedrine), methamphetamine (Desoxyn), and Biphetamine, a mixture of the resins of amphetamine and dextroamphetamine. Also included in this discussion are the nonamphetamine anorexiants phentermine (Ionamin), benzphetamine (Didrex), phenmetrazine (Preludin), phendimetrazine (Plegine), diethylpropion (Tenuate), mazindol (Sanorex), and fenfluramine (Pondimin). They are available in tablets, capsules, and sustained-release preparations.

"Ice" is an illicit crystalline form of methamphetamine that is smoked for instant effects similar to those of intravenous amphetamine.

Mechanism of Toxicity: Amphetamines stimulate the release of norepinephrine and directly stimulate adrenergic receptors. They are direct central nervous system and respiratory stimulants.

Toxic Dose: The toxic dose is not well defined. Symptoms can occur with as little as 5 mg. Doses as low as 1.5 mg/kg have been fatal.

Signs and Symptoms: Central nervous system effects include agitation, confusion, hyperactivity, and delirium. In severe cases, a period of hyperactivity precedes complete collapse. Fasciculations can progress to seizures and coma. Cardiac effects include dysrhythmias, hypertension, cardiomyopathy, and acute myocardial infarction. Hyperpyrexia also has been reported. Pupils may be dilated. Dehydration, rhabdomyolysis, and renal failure have been described. Cerebral hemorrhage and cerebral vasculitis have been described with chronic abuse.

Psychosis and self-destructive behavior is most common following chronic abuse.

Diagnostic Testing: Amphetamines are usually detected in a urine drug screen. Blood levels are not readily available and are not clinically useful.

General Treatment: Because significant symptoms are possible, the need for life-support measures, including cardiac support and seizure precautions, should be anticipated.

Decontamination: (Refer to the treatment section p 6 for the appropriate use of these techniques.) Emesis should be avoided because seizures may occur. Gastric lavage and activated charcoal can be used.

Antidote: No specific antidotes are available.

Specific Treatment: (See Table 3, p 22, for specific dosing.) Seizures can be treated with benzodiazepines. Hypertension usually does not require treatment; short-acting vasodilators such as nitroprusside, however, can be used if necessary. Lidocaine is the preferred agent for managing ventricular dysrhythmias. Hypotension should respond to fluids and pressors. Hyperactivity and agitation usually respond to benzodiazepines. Hyperthermia can be treated with standard therapy. Alkaline diuresis can be used for the treatment of rhabdomyolysis.

Patient Monitoring: Monitor vital signs, mental status, cardiac status, and renal output.

Enhanced Eliminations: Enhanced elimination techniques are of no proven value.

References

Derlet RW, Heischober B. Methamphetamine: stimulant of the 1990s? *West J Med.* 1990;153:625-628

Derlet RW, Rice P, Horowitz BZ, Lord RV. Amphetamine toxicity: experience with 127 cases. *J Emerg Med.* 1989;7:157-161

Hong R, Matsuyama E, Nur K. Cardiomyopathy associated with the smoking of crystal methamphetamine. *JAMA.* 1991;265:1152-1154

Parran TV, Jasinski DR. Intravenous methylphenidate abuse: prototype for prescription drug abuse. *Arch Intern Med.* 1991;151:781-783

Cocaine

Available Forms and Sources: Cocaine is a bitter tasting alkaloid from the leaves of the shrub *Erythroxylon coca*. Available forms of cocaine are the hydrochloride salt, the free base, and "crack." Cocaine hydrochloride is a white powder sold as grams or spoons. A "spoon" is 0.5 g, and a gram can be divided into 30 to 40 lines for insufflation. The typical "line" is 20 to 30 mg. Free-base cocaine is a colorless, odorless, transparent substance that is smoked. Crack usually appears in the form of a light-brown pellet (100 to 150 mg) or a piece of "rock" (300 to 500 mg) and is smoked. Cocaine is used therapeutically as a topical local anesthetic. Pharmaceutical preparations include a powder, soluble tablet, and a solution.

Mechanism of Toxicity: Cocaine stimulates the presynaptic release of dopamine, norepinephrine, serotonin, and acetylcholine in the central nervous system. Long-term use of cocaine can deplete dopamine in the central nervous system and may be the basis for depression and the cycle of chronic addiction.

Toxic Dose: A dose of 50 to 95 mg has been reported to produce psychoactive effects. Cardiac and central nervous system effects may occur at 1 mg/kg.

Signs and Symptoms: The duration of cocaine's action is short, with symptoms occurring over a period of 2 to 3 hours. Signs and symptoms are dose related. Low doses produce euphoria and central nervous system stimulation, while high doses produce anxiety, agitation, paranoid delusions, mydriasis, hypertension, hyperthermia, tachycardia, and cardiac dysrhythmias. Central nervous system stimulation and convulsions are followed by central nervous system and cardiorespiratory depression.

Cardiovascular effects include dysrhythmias that are usually supraventricular, but occasionally ventricular fibrillation and asystole occur. Many cases of myocardial infarction in previously healthy young adults have been temporally related to cocaine abuse.

Neurologic effects include intracerebral hemorrhage and cerebral vasculitis, subarachnoid hemorrhage, and intracranial hemorrhage. Paranoia and paranoid psychosis, formication or incessant scratching at imaginary insects (called "cocaine bugs," or Magnan's sign), suicidal depression, dysphoria, hyperactivity, apprehension, and confusion may develop. Tolerance and psychological addiction develop with repeated use.

Pulmonary complications of cocaine use or abuse include perforation of the nasal septa, pneumomediastinum, pneumothorax, pulmonary edema, alveolar hemorrhage, and bronchiolitis obliterans. Free-base smoking has been associated with reactive airway disease resulting in bronchospasm and recurrent asthmatic episodes. Pulmonary infiltrates ("crack lung") and epiglottitis have also been reported in those who smoke crack.

Intestinal ischemia (cocaine colitis) with hemorrhagic diarrhea and liver dysfunction can occur. Rhabdomyolysis with acute renal failure and priapism can also occur.

Passive inhalation of cocaine may produce seizures and neurological abnormalities in infants and toddlers. Suspect passive cocaine exposure in any new, unexplained seizure in a child. Cocaine is excreted in breast milk and has caused adverse reactions in nursing infants. One infant experienced seizures after nursing from a mother who had applied cocaine to her nipples to ease the pain of nursing.

The reported pregnancy, fetal, and neonatal complications of cocaine abuse are spontaneous abortion, abruptio placenta, intrauterine growth retardation, prematurity, learning disabilities, possible teratogenicity (prune-belly syndrome), increased risk of urogenital anomalies, neonatal cerebral infarction, congenital cardiac defects, arterial thrombosis and hypertension, increased risk of intracranial hemorrhage, and necrotizing enterocolitis. The data on teratogenicity are incomplete, and there is controversy about the existence of a neonatal abstinence syndrome.

A "body packer" or "mule" refers to a person who ingests small packages of contraband to conceal the drug in the gastrointestinal tract during transport. These packages, often condoms, are usually well wrapped and sealed and are designed to withstand prolonged transport. A "body stuffer" refers to a person who ingests substances hastily for the purpose of hiding evidence. The substances are ingested in vials, glassine bags, and sometimes without wrappings. In both body packers and body stuffers, inadvertent leakage or rupture of the package may lead to serious acute toxicity.

Diagnostic Testing: Most drug screens detect cocaine or its metabolites. Cocaine can be detected in urine up to 12 hours after exposure; its metabolite benzoylecognine may be found 48 to 114 hours after exposure, depending on the laboratory method used. Cocaine can be detected in blood but blood levels are not generally available or of clinical value. Herbal teas, lidocaine, and droperidol may give false-positive test results by some laboratory methods. Meconium and hair analysis of newborns is being investigated to identify exposure to cocaine in utero. In infants, passive inhalation may result in a detectable blood level of cocaine.

General Treatment: Because significant symptoms are possible, the need for life support measures should be anticipated.

Decontamination: (Refer to the treatment section p 6 for the appropriate use of these techniques.) Emesis is not recommended. For the more common nonoral routes of exposure, gastrointestinal decontamination is unlikely to be of value because of the small quantities involved and its rapid absorption.

If cocaine is ingested, activated charcoal and a cathartic may be given. Whole bowel irrigation has been used safely to remove packets of cocaine and crack vials in body packers or stuffers. Irrigation is continued until the rectal effluent is clear and the abdominal roentgenogram reveals removal of the packets. If a large ingestion of cocaine has occurred and the initial roentgenogram is normal, a contrast study can confirm successful passage of the drug. Surgical removal of the drug may be indicated if the drug is not in a secure container and does not pass the pylorus.

Cocaine in the nose can be removed with an applicator dipped in a nonwater-soluble product (lubricating jelly).

Antidote: No specific antidotes are available.

Specific Treatment: Control ventricular dysrhythmias with phenytoin. Avoid lidocaine administration because it is often an adulterant of cocaine, can cause seizures, and may enhance cardiac conduction abnormalities. Wide complex dysrhythmias may respond to intravenous sodium bicarbonate to maintain pH at 7.5. Cardioversion should be considered for unstable dysrhythmias. Unstable supraventricular dysrhythmias may be treated by correcting ischemia, calcium channel blockers, α- and β-adrenergic blockers, or cardioversion. Adenosine treatment appears ineffective. Evaluation for myocardial infarction should be considered.

Hypertension may respond to oxygen and diazepam; however, nitroprusside may be necessary to treat severe hypertensive emergencies. Sublingual nifedipine or other calcium channel blockers may be effective. A study using rats, however, indicates that calcium channel blockers may potentiate cocaine toxicity. Labetalol, a β-blocker with weak α-adrenergic action, may also be used. Propranolol should not be used because unopposed alpha action may result in paradoxical hypertension. Esmolol is a short-acting intravenous cardioselective β_1 blocker that has been recommended; however, occasional paradoxical effects occur, and it should not be routinely used.

Control agitation and treat seizures aggressively with diazepam and, if needed, phenytoin. Endotracheal intubation, assisted ventilation, and neuromuscular blockers (with electroencephalogram monitoring for nonmotor seizures) may be needed to control seizures and subsequent lactic acidosis. If neuromuscular blockers are administered, they should be continued until the electroencephalogram is normal for at least 2 hours or more. Haloperidol is not recommended for treatment of agitation.

Manage hyperthermia with vigorous external cooling. Do not use antipyretics. The hyperthermia caused by cocaine toxicity is secondary to hypermetabolism combined with vasoconstriction and alterations in thermoregulation. Dantrolene therapy does not relieve this condition. If rhabdomyolysis is present, alkaline diuresis may be used to avoid precipitation of myoglobin in the renal tubules and renal failure. Increases in enzyme levels due to rhabdomyolysis should be fractionated to differentiate between cardiac and skeletal muscle.

If the patient is pregnant, monitor the fetus and anticipate possible spontaneous abortion or abruptio placenta. If cocaine has been used during pregnancy, ultrasonography for congenital anomalies, especially of the urogenital tract, should be considered.

Patient Monitoring: Obtain a complete blood count, electrocardiogram, levels of cardiac enzymes, and arterial blood gases. If significant neurologic manifestations are present, determine values for blood pH, serum electrolytes, and blood glucose; obtain renal and hepatic profiles, an electroencephalogram, and perform computed tomography.

Enhanced Elimination: Enhanced elimination techniques are of no proven value.

References

Chasnoff IJ, Griffith DR, Freier C, Murray J. Cocaine/polydrug use in pregnancy: two-year followup. *Pediatrics.* 1992;89:284-289

Derlet RW, Albertson TE. Emergency department presentation of cocaine intoxication. *Ann Emerg Med.* 1989;18:182-186

Goldfrank LR, Hoffman RS. The cardiovascular effects of cocaine. *Ann Emerg Med.* 1991;20:165-175

Hoffman RS, Henry GC, Howland MA, Weisman RS, Weil L, Goldfrank LR. Association between life threatening cocaine toxicity and plasma cholinesterase activity. *Ann Emerg Med.* 1992;21:247-253

Kharasch SJ, Glotzer D, Vinci R, Weitzman M, Sargent J. Unsuspected cocaine exposure in young children. *AJDC.* 1991;145:204-206

Rosenberg NM, Meert KL, Knazik SR, Yee H, Kauffman RE. Occult cocaine exposure in children. *AJDC.* 1991;145:1430-1432

Shannon M, Lacouture PG, Roa J, Woolf A. Cocaine exposure among children seen at a pediatric hospital. *Pediatrics.* 1989;83:337-3422

Designer Drugs

Available Forms and Sources: Designer drugs are synthetic analogues of controlled substances produced in an effort to subvert laws governing the possession and distribution of such substances. Although a variety of substances have been synthesized over the years, current popular agents fall into the following three categories: fentanyl analogues, meperidine analogues, and amphetamine analogues.

Fentanyl analogues include α-methylfentanyl (China white or Persian white) and 3-methylfentanyl. Meperidine analogues include MPPP (1-methyl-4-phenyl-4-propionoxypiperidine) and MPTP (1-methyl-4-phenyl-1,2,3,6-tetrahydropyridine). Amphetamine analogues include MDMA (3,4-methylenedioxymethamphetamine; ecstacy, Adam, and XTC), MDA (3,4-methylene-dioxyamphetamine), and MMDA (3-methoxy-4,5-methylene-dioxyamphetamine).

Mechanism of Toxicity: Fentanyl derivatives produce their effect on opioid receptors in the brain, producing an initial "rush" followed by central nervous system depression. MPTP is converted to a toxic metabolite that destroys dopaminergic neurons in the substantia nigra, leading to a parkinsonian-like syndrome. Amphetamine analogues produce hallucinogenic and sympathomimetic effects.

Toxic Dose: The toxic doses of these agents are poorly defined, but are generally thought to be low.

Signs and Symptoms: Fentanyl derivatives generally produce central nervous system depression, which may cause the rapid onset of respiratory arrest. Bradycardia and hypotension may also occur together with hypothermia.

Meperidine analogues are potent central nervous system depressants after acute overdose. The parkinsonian-like syndrome associated with MPTP usually is initially seen with choreiform or extrapyramidal type movement disorders. These symptoms may be irreversible and are thought to be unrelated to dose.

Ingestion of amphetamine analogues, most notably MDMA, has been associated with several deaths. Symptoms are related to the sympathomimetic effects of these drugs—tachycardia, hypertension, severe hyperthermia, and dilated pupils. Bizarre behavior and panic disorders may also be seen.

Diagnostic Testing: These agents usually are not identified on routine drug screens.

General Treatment: Because significant symptoms are possible, the need for cardiorespiratory monitoring and seizure control should be anticipated.

Decontamination: (Refer to the treatment section p 6 for the appropriate use of these techniques.) Emesis is not recommended. Activated charcoal treatment may be of some value.

Because of the small quantities involved and rapid absorption, however, any form of gastric decontamination is of questionable value.

Antidote: Naloxone can be used to reverse the central nervous system and respiratory depressant effects secondary to fentanyl and meperidine derivatives **(see Table 2, p 16, for specific dosing).**

Specific Treatment: Anecdotal reports have described levodopa, bromocriptine, or benztropine for symptomatic treatment of the parkinsonian-like syndrome associated with MPTP toxicity. Patients with this syndrome must be referred to a neurologist for further care.

Patient Monitoring: Patients with significant neurologic or cardiovascular symptoms need intensive monitoring until symptoms resolve.

Enhanced Elimination: Enhanced elimination techniques are of no proven value.

References

Brittain JL. China white: the bogus drug. *J Toxicol Clin Toxicol.* 1982; 19:1123-1126.

Buchanan JF, Brown CR. 'Designer Drugs': a problem in clinical toxicology. *Med Toxicol Adverse Drug Exp.* 1988;3:1-17

Manoguerra AS, Shaw RF, Normann SA. Fentanyl-derivative fatalities in San Diego County. *Vet Hum Toxicol.* 1985;28:295.

Ethanol (Ethyl Alcohol)

Available Forms and Sources: Ethanol is contained in numerous products including liquid cold remedies for adults (2% to 25% ethanol), mouthwashes and plaque rinses (7% to 27%), aftershave lotions (14% to 79%), liniments, tinctures, some rubbing alcohols (70%), perfumes and colognes (25% to 95%), glass cleaners (9% to 10%), and paint remover and stripper (25%). Typical beverages that contain ethanol include whiskey (40% to 50%, or 80 to 100 proof), liqueurs (22% to 50%), wines (10% to 14%), and beer (3% to 8%). The term "proof" defines the alcohol concentration in beverages and is twice the percentage of alcohol.

Mechanism of Toxicity: Ethanol is a general central nervous system depressant and a gastric irritant.

Toxic Dose: An ingested dose of 1 g/kg (about 1 mL/kg of 100% or absolute ethanol) produces a peak blood level of about 100 mg/dL. Blood ethanol levels below 50 mg/dL can produce mild intoxication in children. A lethal dose has been estimated at 3 g/kg equivalent to a blood ethanol level of about 300 mg/dL for children, although young children have survived blood ethanol levels up to 575 mg/dL. A blood ethanol level can be estimated from the dose if it is ingested over a short time (see toxicity calculations, p 28).

Ethanol is well absorbed by inhalation, dermal, or oral routes. Significant dermal and inhalation absorption have been reported after a child was sponged with ethanol to reduce fever.

Signs and Symptoms: Initial exhilaration is followed by incoordination, slurred speech, ataxia, nausea, and vomiting, with risk of aspiration as consciousness is progressively impaired. Increased urination contributes to fluid losses, dehydration, and acidemia. Vasodilation results in flushed skin, sweating, hypothermia, hypotension, and tachycardia. In moderate to severe intoxication, variable pupillary reactions, coma, and shock may occur. Hypoglycemia and seizures can occur in any aged child, but are more common in young children and can occur in relatively mild intoxications. Hypoglycemia occurs more commonly in diabetics.

Diagnostic Testing: Ethanol is detected in most drug screens. Blood ethanol determinations are readily available and are diagnostic. If other alcohols may be present, either immunoassay or gas liquid chromatography is the preferred analytic method. If ethanol alone is suspected, one of the widely used enzymatic assay methods is adequate. Blood ethanol levels generally correlate with symptoms. Performance decrements occur at levels >50 mg/dL.

General Treatment: Because significant symptoms are possible, the need for life support measures including respiratory support should be anticipated.

Decontamination: (Refer to treatment section p 6 for the appropriate use of these techniques.) Emesis should not be induced because of the rapid onset of central nervous system depression. Gastric lavage is likely to be most useful within 30 to 60 minutes after ingestion. Activated charcoal does not bind ethanol and should not be given unless other toxic products have been ingested.

Antidote: (See Table 2, p 16, for specific doses.) There are some reports of reversal of obtundation with naloxone, but the value of this agent is questionable and it is not recommended as an alternative to basic support.

Specific Treatment: Protect the patient against aspiration. Hypoxia may require intubation and mechanical ventilation. Hypoglycemia should be treated with dextrose. Administer intravenous fluids to replace urinary losses and correct electrolyte imbalance, acidemia, and hypotension. Plasma expanders and pressors may be needed to treat severe hypotension. Treat hypothermia and maintain the normal body temperature of the patient. Consider therapy with thiamine (100 mg intravenously or intramuscularly) in any patient who is intoxicated with ethanol, especially older children or adolescents who may be chronic users or abusers.

Patient Monitoring: Monitor serum electrolytes, glucose, serum urea nitrogen, creatinine, and liver transaminase values. An arterial blood gas is helpful to determine the need for ventilatory support in severe intoxication.

Enhanced Elimination: If the blood ethanol level is greater than 300 to 350 mg/dL and clinical deterioration progresses despite supportive treatment, hemodialysis should be instituted.

References

Litovitz T. The alcohols: ethanol, methanol, isopropanol, ethylene glycol. *Pediatr Clin North Am.* 1986;33:311-323

Ricci LR, Hoffman SA. Ethanol-induced hypoglycemic coma in a child. *Ann Emerg Med.* 1982;11:202-204

Scherger DL, Wruk KM, Kulig KW, Rumack BH. Ethyl alcohol (ethanol)-containing cologne, perfume, and after-shave ingestions in children. *AJDC.* 1988;142:630-632

Selbst SM, DeMaio JG, Boenning D. Mouthwash poisoning. *Clin Pediatr.* 1985;24:162-164

Inhalants

Available Forms and Sources: Inhalants come from several different chemical classes. They are commonly abused by children for their mind-altering effects because of their low price, ubiquity, and the lack of legal constraints against their sale to minors. Table 15 lists the most commonly abused inhalants.

Inhalants can be placed into the following three general categories: hydrocarbons, anesthetics, and nitrites. Hydrocarbons include aliphatic hydrocarbons, halogenated hydrocarbons, and other solvents. Nitrous oxide is the only widely abused anesthetic. Several nitrites including isobutyl-, n-butyl-, and amyl nitrite are marketed as room deodorizers.

All of these products are highly volatile and produce mild narcotic effects when inhaled. Additionally, certain inhalants have distinct toxicologic properties (cardiotoxicity or oxidizing potential) that may lead to differing clinical manifestations.

Inhalants may be abused by "huffing," in which a towel is soaked with the inhalant and placed over the nose followed by deep inspiration, or by "bagging," in which the inhalant is placed into a bag or other receptacle that is placed over the face or entire head.

Mechanism of Toxicity: All inhalants are lipophilic, which permits their rapid diffusion into the central nervous system, resulting in altered states of consciousness. This effect is associated with transient euphoria, light-headedness, and feelings of inebri-

Table 15. Commonly Abused Inhalants

Inhalant	Chemical Constituents	Toxicity
Acrylic paint	Toluene	Electrolyte abnormalities
Aerosols, propellants	Fluorocarbons, nitrous oxide, isobutane, helium	Asphyxia
Gasoline	Aliphatics, benzene, organic lead	Lead intoxication
Glues, adhesives	Toluene, benzene, xylene, chlorinated hydrocarbons	Electrolyte abnormalities, cardiac dysrhythmias
Lighter refills	Butane	Asphyxia
Paints, varnishes, lacquers	Trichloroethylene, methylene chloride, toluene	Cardiac dysrhythmias, carbon monoxide poisoning, electrolyte abnormalities
Polystyrene cements	Toluene, hexane, trichloroethylene	Cardiac dysrhythmias
Rubber cement	Benzene, hexane, trichloroethylene	Peripheral neuropathy
Shoe polish	Chlorinated hydrocarbons, toluene	Cardiac dysrhythmias, electrolyte abnormalities
Spot remover	Chlorinated hydrocarbons	Cardiac dysrhythmias
Typewriter correction fluid	Chlorinated hydrocarbons	Cardiac dysrhythmias
Odorizers, "poppers"	Nitrites	Methemoglobinemia

ation. Because inhalants displace oxygen from the immediate environment, they can also act as simple asphyxiants.

Toxic Dose: The toxic dose for these agents via inhalation is not established.

Signs and Symptoms: Each category of inhalant is associated with a different clinical picture after acute or chronic toxicity. Abuse of nitrous oxide may cause asphyxia with acute intoxication but has little established toxicity after chronic abuse. Nitrites are potent oxidizers that produce methemoglobinemia after inhalation.

Several different potential reactions can occur as a result of hydrocarbon toxicity. Halogenated hydrocarbons are myocardial irritants that can cause spontaneous ventricular tachydysrhythmias with acute inhalation. Because hydrocarbons are highly lipid soluble, they readily cross the blood-brain barrier, leading to profound narcosis and central nervous system depression. Hydrocarbons have been associated with "sudden sniffing death," the result of simple asphyxiation, cardiac dysrhythmias, and respiratory arrest from narcosis. Certain hydrocarbons may be metabolized to toxic metabolites (eg, biotransformation of methylene chloride into carbon monoxide). Many hydrocarbons are recognized hepatotoxins. Hydrocarbons may contain toxic constituents that have primary toxicity, eg, lead intoxication from inhalation of leaded gasoline. With chronic use, many hydrocarbons, particularly n-hexane, can lead to peripheral neuropathy. With chronic use, many hydrocarbons cause encephalopathy, the result of a leukoencephalomalacia. Chronic use of aromatic hydrocarbons, particularly toluene, may lead to multisystem dysfunction, which includes muscle wasting, renal tubular acidosis, and profound electrolyte disturbances. Several solvents, particularly benzene, are recognized as possible carcinogens.

Clinical manifestations largely depend on the type of inhalant being abused. Initial signs and symptoms may originate from the nervous system (ataxia, tremor, altered mental status, and dementia), gastrointestinal tract (abdominal pain and anorexia), blood (cyanosis in association with methemoglobinemia), musculoskeletal system (weakness and wasting), or skin (rashes beneath the nares), or they may be entirely nonspecific. With severe intoxication, clinical presentation may be associated with life-threatening coma, asphyxia, cardiac dysrhythmias, or symptomatic methemoglobinemia.

Diagnostic Testing: The clinical diagnosis of inhalant abuse is difficult, although certain features, eg, paint stains or a solvent odor, may be important clues. Urine and serum toxicology screens usually do not detect inhalants.

General Treatment: The patient should be removed from the site of exposure. Provide adequate oxygenation to treat hypoxia. Patients presenting with coma often require respiratory support.

Decontamination: Gastrointestinal decontamination is not necessary due to the route of exposure to these products.

Antidote: No specific antidotes are available.

Specific Treatment: Cardiac disturbances should be treated with standard agents, although epinephrine is theoretically contraindicated because hydrocarbons, particularly halogenated hydrocarbons, sensitize the myocardium to catecholamines, resulting in ventricular irritability and worsening dysrhythmias.

Patient Monitoring: Ancillary tests including an electrocardiogram and determinations of levels of lead in the blood, carboxyhemoglobin, serum creatine phosphokinase, and methemoglobin should be considered depending upon the agent involved. Additionally, a complete metabolic profile including electrolyte levels, liver function tests, and urinalysis should be considered. Cranial tomography should be considered for patients with prolonged alterations in mental status.

Enhanced Elimination: Enhanced elimination techniques are of no proven value.

References

Bass M. Sudden sniffing death. *JAMA*. 1970;212:2075-2079

Flanagan RJ, Ruprah M, Meredity TJ, Ramsey JD. An introduction to the clinical toxicology of volatile substances. *Drug Saf*. 1990;5:359-383

Goldings AS, Stewart RM. Organic lead encephalopathy: behavioral change and movement disorder following gasoline inhalation. *J Clin Psychiatry*. 1982;43:70-71

Hornfeldt CS, Ling LJ, Fifield GC. Inhalation of gasoline fumes. *Clin Pediatr*. 1986;25:114-115

Kulberg A. Substance abuse: clinical identification and management. *Pediatr Clin North Am*. 1986;33:325-361

Morton HG. Occurrence and treatment of solvent abuse in children and adolescents. *Pharmacol Ther*. 1987;33:449-469

Schwartz RH, Peary P. Abuse of isobutyl nitrite inhalation (Rush©) by adolescents. *Clin Pediatr*. 1986;25:308-310

Smart RG. Solvent use in North America: aspects of epidemiology, prevention, and treatment. *J Psychoactive Drugs*. 1986;18:87-96

Troutman WG. Additional deaths associated with the intentional inhalation of typewriter correction fluid. *Vet Hum Toxicol*. 1988;30:130-132

Lysergic Acid Diethylamide (LSD)

Available Forms and Sources: Lysergic acid diethylamide (LSD) is a synthetic ergot alkaloid derivative with no established medical use. It is commonly abused as a hallucinogenic agent. It is sold in tablet, capsule, powder, and liquid forms or impregnated in blotter paper or sugar cubes. Street names include acid, purple haze, white lightening, the beast, sunshine, window pane, and ghost.

Mechanism of Toxicity: Ingestion of LSD is thought to alter serotonin and dopamine activity in the brain. It may also affect the peripheral nervous system.

Toxic Dose: Single oral doses of 30 µg/kg produce significant central nervous system symptoms in adults lasting 24 hours. The lethal adult dose of LSD has been estimated to be 14 mg. Toxic doses in children are not established.

Signs and Symptoms: The most prominent symptoms relate to the central nervous system. Patients often appear anxious and fearful and may exhibit bizarre behavior. They may be combative or self-destructive. Severe intoxication may result in hyperthermia, obtundation, diaphoresis, and hyperreflexia. Rhabdomyolysis also may occur. Cardiac symptoms include tachycardia and either hypotension or hypertension. Flashbacks and acute anxiety attacks have been described with LSD use.

Although a few cases of congenital anomalies have been associated with LSD use during pregnancy, there are no controlled studies demonstrating teratogenicity.

Diagnostic Testing: The diagnosis of LSD ingestion is usually based on history and presenting symptoms. The drug generally is not detected in drug screens. Serum levels of LSD, when available, do not correlate with symptoms.

General Treatment: Treatment is generally supportive. Because the usual cause of death is trauma, patients must be protected from self-injury.

Decontamination: (Refer to the treatment section p 6 for the appropriate use of these techniques.) Emesis is not recommended. Lavage is unlikely to be effective because of the small dose ingested. Activated charcoal can be administered.

Antidote: No specific antidotes are available.

Specific Treatment: (See Table 3, p 22, for specific dosing.) Anxiety and agitation are best treated with sensory isolation and reassurance. If a pharmacologic agent is needed, diazepam or midazolam are the agents of choice. Antipsychotic agents should be avoided because of the risk of seizures or hypotension.

Patient Monitoring: Monitor vital signs and cardiac and mental status.

Enhanced Elimination: Enhanced elimination techniques are of no proven value.

References

Friedman SA, Hirsch SE. Extreme hypothermia after LSD ingestion. *JAMA.* 1971;217:1549-1550

Ianzito BM, Liskow B, Stewart MA. Reaction to LSD in a two-year-old child. *J Pediatr.* 1972;80:643-647

Margolis S, Martin L. Anophthalmia in an infant of parents using LSD. *Ann Ophthamol.* 1980;12:1378-1381

Samuelsson BO. LSD intoxication in a two-year-old child. *Acta Paediatr Scand.* 1974;63:797-798

Wason S. LSD intoxication. *Ann Emerg Med.* 1985;14:487

Marijuana

Available Forms and Sources: Marijuana is the dried, cut foliage of the annual herb *Cannabis sativa*. The major active constituent is delta-9-tetrahydrocannabinol (Δ^9-THC). It is usually smoked for its psychotomimetic effect, although symptoms may also follow ingestion. Hashish is a dried resin from the same plant containing a higher percentage of Δ^9-THC. Street names include Mary Jane, pot, MJ, and grass.

Mechanism of Toxicity: The exact mechanism of action of marijuana is not known. The two primary target organs are the central nervous system and the cardiovascular system.

Toxic Dose: The estimated lethal dose of cannabis is 30 mg/kg of absorbed active ingredients. Most marijuana plants grown in the United States contain 1% to 6% Δ^9-THC. Thus, a 500-mg cigarette usually contains 5 to 30 mg, which produces short-lived euphoria when smoked in most persons. Ingestion of marijuana cigarettes has lead to coma in young children.

Signs and Symptoms: Smoking or ingesting marijuana usually produces a state of euphoria and relaxation. It is claimed to heighten sensory awareness. Smoking marijuana compromises the ability to perform complex psychological and motor tasks such as driving. High doses may cause paranoid behavior or psychosis with hallucinations and bizarre behavior. Coma may occur following large ingestions in small children.

The heart rate is generally increased with increased cardiac output, leading to reddened conjunctivae. Large doses may produce postural hypotension.

Inhalation of marijuana leads to bronchodilation. Chronic smoking may lead to bronchitis. Marijuana smoke is thought to be more carcinogenic than tobacco smoke. There are no well-described cases of death from smoking or ingesting marijuana.

Marijuana use during pregnancy has been associated with prematurity, lower birth weight, and congenital features similar to those of fetal alcohol syndrome. Whether these findings represent true teratogenicity or only concomitant alcohol abuse in smokers is unclear. Delta-9-THC concentrates in breast milk.

Long-term, heavy usage of marijuana can lead to tolerance and physical dependence and has been associated with decreased sperm counts and abnormal morphologic features in sperm.

Diagnostic Testing: The biologically inactive metabolite of Δ^9-THC, 11-Nor-Δ^9-tetrahydrocannabinol-9-carboxylic acid (9-carboxy-THC) is detected in most urine drug screens. Test results that indicate the presence of this metabolite require confirmation by a more specific method if necessary. Positive urine screens only reflect prior usage and they do not correlate with clinical effects. Marijuana use may be detected up to several days following the smoking of a single cigarette and up to 4 weeks after the last exposure in chronic users. Passive exposure to marijuana smoke rarely is detected by urine testing. Serum levels of Δ^9-THC can be measured; they do not, however, correlate well with clinical effects and generally are not useful.

General Treatment: Marijuana exposure rarely requires medical intervention except in the cases of large ingestion by children.

Decontamination: **(Refer to the treatment section p 6 for the appropriate use of these techniques.)** Emesis should not be induced because of the possibility of coma. Gastric lavage may not be effective at removing plant material. Activated charcoal is the treatment of choice if gastric decontamination is required and less than 4 to 6 hours has elapsed since ingestion.

Antidote: No specific antidotes are available.

Specific Treatment: **(See Table 3, p 22, for specific dosing.)** Hypotension can be treated with intravenous fluids and pressors as necessary. Extreme agitation can be treated with benzodiazepines if necessary.

Patient Monitoring: Monitor mental status and vital signs.

Enhanced Elimination: Enhanced elimination techniques are of no proven value.

References

Hingson R, Alpert JJ, Day N, Dooling E. Effects of maternal drinking and marijuana use on fetal growth and development. *Pediatrics.* 1982;70:539-546

Relman AS. Marijuana and health. *N Engl J Med.* 1982;306:603-605

Weinberg D, Lande A, Hilton N, Kerns DL. Intoxication from accidental marijuana ingestion. *Pediatrics.* 1983;71:848-850

Methaqualone

Available Forms and Sources: Methaqualone is a lipid-soluble nonbarbiturate sedative-hypnotic that was withdrawn from the American market in 1984. Illicit sources remain available, but commonly contain adulterants or alternate substances. In 1983, only 32% of the drug samples alleged to be methaqualone contained the unadulterated drug. Frequent additives or substitutes include diazepam, phencyclidine, or barbiturates.

Mechanism of Toxicity: Pharmacological activity is primarily due to central nervous system depression. The anticonvulsant activity is mediated by serotonin pathways in the brain. Other activities include antispasmodic, local anesthetic, and antihistaminic effects. An increase in vascular permeability increases the likelihood of pulmonary edema. Some of the adverse reactions may be related to impurities in street sources, such as ortho-toluidine, which causes hemorrhagic cystitis.

Toxic Dose: Although oral doses of 8 to 20 g (100 to 200 mg/kg) have caused death in adults, others have survived ingestions of as much as 24 g (>300 mg/kg). Large amounts of alcohol were also ingested in some fatal cases. A correlation exists between dose, severity of symptoms, and the duration of sedation. An average dose of 2.4 g produces coma. Tolerance occurs with chronic abuse and affects the toxic dose. The toxic dose in children is not well defined.

Signs and Symptoms: With low toxic doses (40 to 80 mg/kg), symptoms are similar to those of other sedatives; dizziness, ataxia, slurred speech, drowsiness, nystagmus, nausea, vomiting, and epigastric discomfort have been reported. At higher doses, increased muscle tone, agitation, increased motor activity, myoclonus, and tonic convulsions are usually seen. Deep tendon reflexes may be increased.

Respiratory depression is exhibited by poor ventilation, although the respiratory rate may be normal or increased. The cough reflex may be diminished. Blood pressure generally is normal. In severe poisoning (>200 mg/kg), deep coma, hypotension (usually mild), tachycardia, oliguria, hemorrhage (gastrointestinal, retinal, or dermal), toxic liver reactions, respiratory depression, apnea, and cerebral and pulmonary edema have been reported. Coma has been reported to last 4 to 96 hours with supportive care. Upward plantar reflexes and polyneuropathy have been reported. Tonic seizures are associated with a dysrhythmic pattern on an electroencephalogram. Pupils are dilated and fixed, and vertical disconjugate eye movements may mimic brain lesions. Both hypothermia and hyperthermia may develop, but hyperthermia may be a sign of aspiration pneumonia.

Thrombocytopenia and prothrombin time (PT) prolongation have been reported. Fixed drug eruptions, erythema multiforme, and urticaria may occur after abuse; adulterants may be responsible for this reaction.

Diagnostic Testing: Methaqualone is detected in most routine drug screens. Plasma levels are not readily available and do not correlate well with toxicity. Levels greater than 9 µg/mL are associated with coma. The therapeutic range is 1 to 5 µg/mL, the toxic range is 10 to 30 µg/mL, and the drug is generally lethal at levels >30 µg/mL.

General Treatment: Because significant symptoms are possible, the need for life support measures including respiratory support and maintenance of fluid and electrolyte balance and urine output should be anticipated.

Decontamination: (Refer to the treatment section p 6 for the appropriate use of these techniques.) Due to the rapid onset of sedation, emesis is contraindicated. Gastric lavage with activated charcoal or activated charcoal treatment alone should be considered if a potentially toxic dose has been ingested.

Antidote: No specific antidotes are available.

Specific Treatment: (See Table 3, p 22, for specific dosing.) Treat tonic seizures with benzodiazepines. If the toxicity is severe, neuromuscular blockade with supportive ventilation may be required. Vasopressors (dopamine or norepinephrine) may be administered following fluid challenge for hypotension.

Patient Monitoring: In patients with significant intoxication, monitor liver and renal function; obtain a complete blood count, partial thromboplastin time (PTT), prothrombin time (PT), an electrocardiogram, and arterial blood gases; and determine levels of platelets, electrolytes, and glucose.

Enhanced Elimination: Forced diuresis is contraindicated because it may precipitate pulmonary edema. Peritoneal dialysis is not of value. Hemodialysis or hemoperfusion may be used in life-threatening situations because, although large amounts of the drug may not be cleared, accelerated clinical improvement has been reported.

References

Abboud RT, Freedman MT, Rogers RM, Daniele RP. Methaqualone poisoning with muscular hyperactivity necessitating the use of curare. *Chest.* 1974;65:204-205

Majelyne W, DeClerck F, Demeter J, Heyndrickx A. Treatment evaluation of a severe methaqualone intoxication in man. *Vet Hum Toxicol.* 1979;21(suppl):201-204

Matthew H, Proudfoot AT, Brown SS, Smith AC. Mandrax poisoning: conservative management of 116 patients. *Br Med J.* 1968;2:101-102

Slazinski L, Knox DW. Fixed drug eruption due to methaqualone. *Arch Dermatol.* 1984;120:1073-1075

Phencyclidine (PCP)

Available Forms and Sources: Phencyclidine (PCP), formerly used as a veterinary anesthetic, is no longer legally available in the United States. However, it is easily manufactured and readily available illicitly in many areas. It is commonly sold as a white crystalline powder, although it may be colored and may be sold as tablets or capsules, impregnated on paper, or mixed with marijuana. It is usually smoked, but it may be insufflated or ingested. Common street names include angel dust, peace, hog, rocket fuel, crystal, and surfer.

Mechanism of Toxicity: Phencyclidine is pharmacologically classed as a dissociative anesthetic. It presumably effects the levels of several neurotransmitters.

Toxic Dose: The effects after a dose are highly variable. The usual dose required to produce the desired central nervous system effect is 1 to 20 mg. Doses greater than 100 mg may be severely toxic.

Signs and Symptoms: The effects of PCP are highly dependent on dose, route of administration, and individual variability. At lower doses distorted behavior and thought patterns predominate. Bizarre and violent behavior, coupled with sensory anesthesia, may be very difficult to control. At high doses vomiting, hypersalivation, hypertension, muscle rigidity, and catatonia may be seen. Sedation is common in young children. Very large doses, particularly by ingestion, may lead to coma with respiratory depression, seizures, opisthotonos, and decerebrate rigidity. Rhabdomyolysis may occur. Death is rare and is usually due to trauma or drowning. Tolerance may develop with chronic use but physical addiction does not occur. Maternal use during pregnancy may be teratogenic and may produce withdrawal symptoms in the infant.

Diagnostic Testing: PCP is not detected in most routine drug screens. Levels of PCP in the blood are low, difficult to measure, and do not correlate well with symptoms. The drug concentrates in gastric fluid and urine and is therefore more easily detected in these fluids.

General Treatment: Treatment is primarily supportive. The patient should be protected from self-inflicted injury.

Decontamination: (Refer to the treatment section p 6 for the appropriate use of these techniques.) Emesis is contraindicated because the risk of aspiration is significant. Gastric lavage is unlikely to be effective because of the small quantity of material ingested. Activated charcoal may be administered.

Antidote: No specific antidotes are available.

Specific Treatment: (See Table 3, p 22, for specific dosing.) Diazepam and haloperidol are the preferred sedative agents if sensory isolation is not adequate. Phenothiazines should not be administered because they may produce hypotension. Elevated blood pressure is usually of short duration and does not require treatment; nitroprusside or diazoxide can be administered if necessary.

Patient Monitoring: Urine should be monitored for hematuria and myoglobinuria. Monitor vital signs and mental status.

Enhanced Elimination: Repeat doses of activated charcoal increase the elimination of PCP, which recycles through the gastrointestinal tract. Continuous gastric suction may also be useful in removing drug concentrated in this gastric fluid. Dialytic techniques are not clinically useful.

References

McCarron MM, Schulze BW, Thompson GA, Conder MC, Goetz WA. Acute phencyclidine intoxication: incidence of clinical findings in 1000 cases. *Ann Emerg Med.* 1981;10:237-242

Schwartz RH, Einhorn A. PCP intoxication in seven young children. *Pediatr Emerg Care.* 1986;2:238-241

Strauss AA, Modaniou HD, Bosu SK. Neonatal manifestations of maternal phencyclidine (PCP) abuse. *Pediatrics.* 1981;68:550-552

CHEMICALS

Alkalis and Acids

Available Forms and Sources: Alkaline materials are found in oven cleaners, drain cleaners, electric dishwasher detergents, Clinitest tablets, laundry detergents, industrial-strength bleach, disc batteries, and denture cleaners. Alkalis include sodium hydroxide, potassium hydroxide, trisodium phosphate, wood ash lye, sodium or potassium carbonate, calcium oxide, and ammonium hydroxide (ammonia). Pure or concentrated products occur as liquids, powders, crystals, or compressed beads. Acids are found in toilet bowl cleaners, soldering fluxes, automobile battery fluid, slate cleaners, and antirust compounds. Acids include hydrofluoric, phosphoric, sulfuric, hydrochloric, and oxalic.

Mechanism of Toxicity: Alkalis produce liquefactive necrosis with penetrating tissue injury and risk of perforation. Acids produce coagulation necrosis with a lower perforation risk.

Toxic Dose: The caustic action of alkalis and acids depends on the concentration of free base or acid at the mucosal, conjunctival, or skin surface. The severity of the burn is determined by the concentration, contact time, and pH (<2 or >12 are potentially more serious) of the product. One crystal of an alkaline drain cleaner can produce a serious burn. Solid alkalis may adhere to the mucosal surface and cause deep injury to the esophagus. Liquids produce a more superficial, often circumferential burn. Alkalis tend to burn the mouth and esophagus more frequently than the stomach; acids often injure all three areas. The absence of oral burns does not exclude esophageal damage, and oral burns do not always indicate esophageal damage.

Signs and Symptoms: Oral burns often manifest as whitish lesions with associated burning pain. Retrosternal pain, salivation, dysphagia, and vomitus containing mucous and blood indicate esophageal injury. Examination of the esophagus by endoscopy demonstrates erythema, edema, ulceration, and necrosis.

Shock may develop. Death may result from shock, aspiration that causes fulminant tracheitis or pneumonia, or glottic edema. After 2 to 4 days of apparent improvement, sudden pain in the abdomen or chest and shock may indicate perforation of the stomach or esophagus. Esophageal stricture may develop following alkali injury and acids may produce gastric outlet obstruction. Dermal and ocular burns also may occur.

Diagnostic Testing: These compounds are not detected in a routine drug screen. See the Specific Treatment section below for a discussion of endoscopy.

General Treatment: Because severe symptoms are possible, the need for life-support measures, including respiratory support, should be anticipated following significant ingestions.

Decontamination: (**Refer to the treatment section p 6 for the appropriate use of these techniques.**) Oral, ocular, and dermal decontamination should be instituted rapidly to decrease the length of contact time with the offending agent. Irrigate eyes with tepid water for at least 15 minutes. Remove contaminated clothing and irrigate the skin with tepid water for 15 minutes. DO NOT attempt to neutralize the alkali or acid.

After ingestion, do not induce vomiting or perform gastric lavage. Rinse the agent out of the patient's mouth and give a few sips of clear fluid if he or she can swallow. Nothing else should be given by mouth. Activated charcoal should not be used.

Antidote: No specific antidotes are available.

Specific Treatment: If a significant ingestion is suspected, promptly consult an endoscopist. The timing of esophagoscopy to determine the extent of corrosive damage varies. Some believe it should be done 12 to 24 hours after ingestion. Others believe a delay of 48 to 72 hours allows edema to subside to enable a more thorough examination. Examinations should not be done after 72 hours due to the risk of perforation. Endoscopy confirms the presence, depth (first-, second-, or third-degree burn), and circumferential nature of the injury. Injury of the muscle layer (third-degree burn) or circumferential burns increase the likelihood of stricture.

In the acute stage of injury, a barium swallow does not yield useful information, but 7 to 10 days after injury, it can confirm the absence of a significant burn. Serial esophagrams should be obtained to monitor for stricture formation in patients with significant injury. Tracheostomy is indicated when obstruction occurs secondary to laryngeal edema. Chest and abdominal roentgenograms confirm aspiration or perforation, if suspected. Circulation should be maintained with fluids or plasma.

The use of broad-spectrum antibiotics is controversial, but is generally indicated only with clear superimposed infection. Recent evidence indicates that steroids do not prevent stricture formation following third-degree burns. First- and second-degree esophageal injuries heal without stricture formation with or without steroid treatment. Current evidence does not support steroid use for either alkali or acid ingestions. Esophageal stricture or gastric outlet obstruction may require subsequent dilation and bougienage or surgical reconstruction. Hydrofluoric acid dermal burns are treated with calcium gluconate used topically, by local injection, or intra-arterially **(see Table 3, p 22, for specific dosing).**

Patient Monitoring: Electrolyte levels should be monitored following significant exposures to alkalis and acids. Arterial blood gases must be monitored if pulmonary symptoms develop.

Enhanced Elimination: Enhanced elimination techniques are of no proven value.

References

Anderson KD, Rouse TM, Randolph JG. A controlled trial of corticosteroids in children with corrosive injury of the esophagus. *N Engl J Med.* 1990;323:637-640

Friedman EM, Lovejoy FH Jr. The emergency management of caustic ingestions. *Emerg Med Clin North Am.* 1984;2:77-86

Gaudreault P, Parent M, McGuigan MA, Chicoine L, Lovejoy FH Jr. Predictability of esophageal injury from signs and symptoms: a study of caustic ingestion in 378 children. *Pediatrics.* 1983;71:767-770

Howell JM. Alkaline ingestions. *Ann Emerg Med.* 1986;15:820-825

Penner GE. Acid ingestion: toxicology and treatment. *Ann Emerg Med.* 1980;9:374-379

Wason S. The emergency management of caustic ingestions. *J Emerg Med.* 1985;2:175-182

Arsenic

Available Forms and Sources: Arsenic is available as inorganic and organic compounds in trivalent and pentavalent oxidation states. Sources of arsenic include pesticides, industry, and environmental contamination.

Mechanism of Toxicity: Arsenic interacts with sulfhydryl groups of proteins and enzymes and substitutes for phosphorus in a variety of biochemical reactions. These interactions inhibit various mitochondrial enzymes and uncouple oxidative phosphorylation, resulting in the impairment of cellular respiration.

Toxic Dose: The toxicity of arsenic compounds varies with their physical and chemical properties. Absorption of arsenicals may occur by inhalation, ingestion, or percutaneously following prolonged contact. The extent of absorption from the gastrointestinal tract can be generalized by the following relationship.

Inorganic arsenicals > Organic arsenicals

Arsenates > Arsenites > Arsenic trioxide

Arsenites (trivalent arsenicals) are more toxic than arsenates (pentavalent arsenicals). In a small child, toxicity may occur following exposure to just milligram amounts of available arsenic.

Signs and Symptoms: Signs and symptoms of acute and chronic arsenic poisoning are generally nonspecific and may closely resemble many natural disease states.
Acute arsenic poisoning. Gastroenteritis is commonly reported following acute arsenic ingestion. The onset of toxicity may be evident within minutes after ingestion, or may be delayed for several hours if food is present in the stomach. Gastrointestinal effects may include metallic taste, garlic odor on the breath, dysphagia, severe nausea, projectile vomiting, abdominal pain,

watery or bloody diarrhea, and dehydration with intense thirst. Central nervous system effects may include drowsiness and confusion, psychosis, muscle cramps, convulsions, coma, and death due to shock. Painful paresthesias of the hands and feet along with a progressive distal muscle weakness may develop several days after ingestion.

Other findings following a severe poisoning may include cold and clammy skin, fluid and electrolyte disturbances, hypovolemia from capillary leaking (third-spacing of fluids), some degree of circulatory collapse, electrocardiographic changes, pulmonary edema, respiratory failure, hemolysis, and renal damage.

Chronic arsenic poisoning. The effects of chronic arsenic poisoning may include a variety of skin and nail changes, diarrhea, chronic malabsorption, hepatic damage, symmetric polyneuropathy involving both sensory and motor neurons in a stocking-glove distribution, muscular weakness of the extremities with eventual paralysis and muscle wasting, encephalopathy, renal damage, hematologic abnormalities, cardiac conduction abnormalities, and peripheral vascular system damage.

Diagnostic Testing: Arsenic is not detected in most drug screens. Arsenic is radiopaque, and an abdominal roentgenogram is suggested if arsenic ingestion is suspected. For symptomatic patients, obtain 24-hour urinary arsenic levels and blood arsenic levels.

A 24-hour urinary arsenic level (chelated or nonchelated) exceeding 50 μg/24 h is usually abnormal. Ingestion of seafood (particularly shellfish) can cause transient elevation of urinary arsenic concentrations. A blood arsenic concentration of less than 7 μg/dL is considered in the normal range.

General Treatment: Begin fluid repletion as soon as possible. Treat shock with oxygen, blood, and fluids as needed.

Decontamination: (Refer to the treatment section p 6 for the appropriate use of these techniques.) Emesis is generally not recommended. Gastric lavage can be performed if instituted early. Whole bowel irrigation should be considered if a roentgenogram demonstrates arsenic in the lower gastrointestinal tract. Activated charcoal may not bind significant amounts of arsenic; however, its administration is recommended until definitive quantitative data on its efficacy are available.

Antidote: The treatment of choice for arsenic poisoning is chelation therapy using BAL in oil (dimercaprol). Chelation therapy should continue until the 24-hour urinary arsenic concentration is less than 50 μg/24 h. An oral chelator such as d-penicillamine or succimer may be substituted when the patient's condition has stabilized or symptoms have resolved **(see Table 2, p 16, for specific dosing).**

Specific Treatment: Correct dehydration and electrolyte abnormalities. Maintain blood pressure with fluids or vasopressors. Tachycardia, usually a response to hypovolemia, should be treated initially with fluid replacement. Ventricular tachycardia or ventricular fibrillation should be treated with standard therapy.

Patient Monitoring: Obtain a complete blood count and urinalysis, and perform electrolyte, liver, and renal function tests. Monitor the electrocardiogram, intravascular fluid status, and vital signs (especially blood pressure).

Enhanced Elimination: Hemodialysis will remove arsenic. Evidence, however, indicates that renal clearance in patients without renal insufficiency is more efficient than hemodialysis.

References

Graziano JH, Cuccia D, Friedheim E. The pharmacology of 2,3-dimercaptosuccinic acid and its potential use in arsenic poisoning. *J Pharmacol Exp Ther.* 1978;207:1051-1055

Malachowski ME. An update on arsenic. *Clin Lab Med.* 1990;10:459-472

Mathieu D, Mathieu-Nolf M, Germain-Alonso M, Neviere R, Furon D, Wattel F. Massive arsenic poisoning—effect of hemodialysis and dimercaprol on arsenic kinetics. *Intensive Care Med.* 1992;18:47-50

Peterson RG, Rumack BH. d-Penicillamine therapy of acute arsenic poisoning. *J Pediatr.* 1977;91:661-666

Asbestos

Available Forms and Sources: Asbestos refers to a group of naturally occurring silicate minerals with a fibrous structure. Types of asbestos include amosite, crocidolite, chrysotile, and tremolite.

It is estimated that about 10 000 schools built during 1946 to 1973 may contain asbestos. Levels of contamination in schools may range from 0.2 fibers per cubic centimeter of air down to 0.05 or less compared to the Occupational Safety and Health Administration (OSHA) workplace standard of 2 fibers per cubic centimeter of air.

Mechanism of Toxicity: The actual molecular mechanism of toxicity of asbestos is unknown. Amosite and crocidolite are cleared more slowly from the lungs than is chrysotile and are more strongly associated with the development of mesothelioma than is chrysotile. Crocidolite is more strongly associated with development of lung cancer than is chrysotile. The latency period for development of disease is many years. Exposure during childhood is thought to predispose to adulthood disease. Cigarette smoking markedly increases the risk for disease. High concentrations of asbestos dust can be severely irritating to the lungs.

Signs and Symptoms: The signs and symptoms of pulmonary malignancy include the gradual development (usually in adults) of dyspnea and cough, with or without sputum production, fatigue, weight loss, and chest pain—all relatively nonspecific. In advanced disease, expansion of the thorax is limited and inspiratory crackles, clubbing of the digits, and cyanosis of the extremities are found. Chest roentgenograms show fibrosis of the lungs, especially in the lower lobes.

Diagnostic Testing: Presence of a history of exposure (usually occupational), physical findings, and evidence on a chest roentgenogram often are adequate to make the diagnosis. A knowledge of or a suspicion of a history of exposure is most important. When needed, a pulmonary biopsy may be indicated. Hallmarks for a histologic diagnosis include discrete foci of fibrosis in the respiratory bronchiolar walls with the presence of asbestos bodies, ferruginous bodies (fibers coated with hemosiderin and glycoproteins), or both. Asbestos is not detected in a drug screen.

General Treatment: No specific treatment is known at this time. Prevention of exposure is the most important measure.

Decontamination: Gastrointestinal decontamination is not necessary.

Specific Treatment: Treatment is supportive. There is no specific treatment.

Patient Monitoring: No specific monitoring is necessary.

Enhanced Elimination: Enhanced elimination techniques are not necessary.

References

Becklake MR. Exposure to asbestos and human disease. *N Engl J Med.* 1982;306:1480-1482

Council on Scientific Affairs. A physician's guide to asbestos-related diseases. *JAMA.* 1984;252:2593-2597

Craighead JE, Mossman BT. The pathogenesis of asbestos-associated diseases. *N Engl J Med.* 1982;306:1446-1455

Mossman BT, Gee JB. Asbestos-related diseases. *N Engl J Med.* 1989;320:1721-1730

Spooner CM. Asbestos in schools: a public health problem. *N Engl J Med.* 1979;301:782-783

Bleach

Available Forms and Sources: Common household bleach usually contains sodium hypochlorite in a 5% to 6% solution, with a pH of about 11.4. Other bleaches include industrial products containing sodium peroxide, sodium perborate, sodium carbonate, and oxalic acid. Many of these products have a higher pH and concentration and are more caustic. Five percent calcium hypochlorite, a mildew remover, is much more caustic than ordinary household bleach.

Mechanism of Toxicity: Because these products are caustic, they have the potential to injure the tissues of the oropharynx, esophagus, stomach, and eye, producing clinical states that vary from mild irritation to corrosion. The degree of damage depends on the amount ingested, the physical form of the product, the duration of exposure, the pH, and the concentration or causticity of the product.

Toxic Dose: A single swallow of household bleach produces only minor symptoms. More significant symptoms may occur following a swallow of industrial-strength bleach products.

Signs and Symptoms: These substances are remarkable emetics, and almost all children who ingest relatively small amounts vomit soon after ingestion. Abdominal pain may develop. Oropharyngeal, esophageal, and gastric burns are unlikely following ingestion of most of these products. An immediate burning sensation occurs after ocular exposure, followed by erythema, lacrimation, edema, and photophobia, but these injuries are rarely serious.

Mixing bleach with ammonia generates chloramine gas (see p 177). Mixing a hypochlorite bleach with an acid, such as a toilet bowl cleaner, generates chlorine gas (see p 179).

Diagnostic Testing: These agents are not detected on a routine drug screen.

General Treatment: Do not attempt to neutralize these agents, which are usually alkaline, because the chemical reaction could cause an exothermic response that can further harm the tissues involved.

Decontamination: (Refer to the treatment section p 6 for the appropriate use of these techniques.) Emesis or gastric lavage is contraindicated. Activated charcoal should not be used. Rinse exposed eyes with water. For dermal exposures, remove clothing and rinse skin thoroughly.

Antidote: No specific antidotes are available.

Specific Treatment: Esophagoscopy is generally not indicated following household bleach ingestion. If the patient is drooling, unable to swallow, or pain persists, esophagoscopy should be considered.

Patient Monitoring: No specific monitoring is necessary.

Enhanced Elimination: Enhanced elimination techniques are of no proven value.

References

Friedman EM, Lovejoy FH. The emergency management of caustic ingestions. *Emerg Med Clin North Am.* 1984;2:77-86

Landau GD, Saunders WH. The effect of chlorine bleach on the esophagus. *Arch Otolaryngol.* 1964;80:174-176

Pike DG, Peabody JW, Davis EW, Lyons WS. A reevaluation of the dangers of Clorox ingestion. *J Pediatr.* 1963;63:303-305

Reisz GR, Gammon RS. Toxic pneumonitis from mixing household cleaners. *Chest.* 1986;89:49-52

Carbon Monoxide

Available Forms and Sources: Carbon monoxide (CO) is produced when any carbon-containing material such as wood, oil, gasoline, or natural gas is burned. Carbon dioxide is also produced. The relative proportions of these two products of combustion depend upon the amount of oxygen available, with limited oxygen favoring the production of carbon monoxide. Carbon monoxide is also a product of the metabolism of methylene chloride. Very small amounts of CO are produced naturally by the catabolism of hemoglobin in the body.

Mechanism of Toxicity: Carbon monoxide toxicity results from several mechanisms. The relative importance of these effects in vivo is not clear. Carbon monoxide binds to hemoglobin with an affinity 250 times greater than oxygen. Relatively small concentrations (<0.5%) of CO in inhaled air can dramatically alter the body's ability to transport oxygen. It also impairs the ability of hemoglobin bound to oxygen to release oxygen to the tissues. Finally, CO binds to cytochrome oxidase, adversely affecting the ability of tissues to utilize oxygen.

Toxic Dose: Toxicity depends upon the amount of CO reaching the circulation, which is determined by the concentration of CO in air and the duration of exposure. Exposure to >0.5% CO for only a few minutes can be lethal, while exposure to >0.15% for longer than an hour may also be lethal.

Signs and Symptoms: The signs and symptoms of CO poisoning relative to carboxyhemoglobin (HbCO) levels are shown in Table 16. Infants and young children are somewhat more sensitive to CO than older children and adults and may experience more severe symptoms at any HbCO level. Signs and symptoms do not always correlate well with measured HbCO levels, probably reflecting the multiple mechanisms of CO poisoning.

Table 16. Carbon Monoxide Blood Levels Versus Signs and Symptoms

HbCO Level, %	Signs and Symptoms
0-10	Most people are asymptomatic. Mild headache, decreased exercise tolerance. May impair driving skills.
10-20	Headache (often temporal and throbbing), fatigue, and nausea
20-30	Severe headache, syncope, dizziness, visual changes, weakness, nausea, vomiting
30-40	Headache, syncope, confusion, loss of consciousness, tachycardia, nausea, vomiting, leukocytosis
40-50	Coma, convulsions, tachycardia, tachypnea
50-60	Coma, convulsions, shock, Cheyne-Stokes respirations, apnea
>60	Death from cardiorespiratory collapse possible

A small percentage of patients with significant CO exposure develop delayed (2 to 40 days) neurological deficits including mental and personality changes, gait disturbances, incontinence, and mutism. Evidence suggests that aggressive treatment may diminish the risk of these symptoms, which may be permanent.

Diagnostic Testing: If CO poisoning is suspected, a carboxyhemaglobin (HbCO) level should be obtained. A low level does not rule out poisoning if the measurement is obtained several hours after termination of the exposure or if oxygen has been administered prior to obtaining the sample. Arterial blood gases may be normal. Oxygen saturation will be low if it is measured rather than calculated.

General Treatment: General supportive therapy, including the administration of 100% oxygen via a non-rebreathing mask or endotracheal tube, is the mainstay of treatment.

Decontamination: Remove the victim to fresh air and begin oxygen therapy as soon as possible.

Antidote: No specific antidotes are available.

Specific Treatment: For patients with major exposures, the use of hyperbaric oxygen (HBO) should be considered, if available. The half-life of CO is approximately 4 to 6 hours in room air but is shortened to about 1 hour in 100% oxygen and to 20 to 30 minutes in HBO (3 atm). The indications for HBO treatment are a carboxyhemaglobin concentration of >25% to 30% (lower if the patient is pregnant); major symptoms, including loss of consciousness, seizures, or cardiac dysrhythmias; or other symptoms unresponsive to 100% oxygen therapy.

Limited data indicate that HBO may prevent the development of delayed neurologic sequelae. There are also anecdotal reports of successful treatment of delayed neurological sequelae with HBO. Additional data are needed to assess the value of HBO in the latter situation.

Patient Monitoring: Levels of HbCO should be monitored during and at the end of therapy. Other monitoring is dictated by patient symptoms.

Enhanced Elimination: Enhanced elimination techniques other than HBO are of no value.

References

Caravati EM, Adams CJ, Joyce SM, Schafer NC. Fetal toxicity associated with maternal carbon monoxide poisoning. *Ann Emerg Med.* 1988;17:714-717

Ginsberg MD. Carbon monoxide intoxication: clinical features, neuropathology and mechanisms of injury. *J Toxicol Clin Toxicol.* 1985;23:281-288

Hampson NB, Norkook DM. Carbon monoxide poisoning in children riding in the back of pickup trucks. *JAMA.* 1992;267:538-540

Lacey DJ. Neurologic sequelae of acute carbon monoxide intoxication. *AJDC.* 1981;135:145-147

Longo LD. The biological effects of carbon monoxide on the pregnant woman, fetus and newborn infant. *Am J Obstet Gynecol.* 1977;129:69-103

Mofenson HC, Caraccio TR, Brody GM. Carbon monoxide poisoning. *Am J Emerg Med.* 1984;2:254-261

Myers RA, Snyder SK, Emhoff TA. Subacute sequelae of carbon monoxide poisoning. *Ann Emerg Med.* 1985;14:1163-1167

Chloramine Gas

Available Forms and Sources: Mixing ammonia with sodium hypochlorite (bleach) produces monochloramine (NH_2Cl), dichloramine ($NHCl_2$), and nitrogen trichloride (NCl_3) gases. The addition of bleach to other sources of urea or ammonia, such as in toilets with standing urine or sewage storage tanks, can also produce chloramine. The combination of acids with hypochlorite/ammonia mixtures enhances formation of chloramine. Since the 1979 Environmental Protection Agency regulation of trihalomethane levels in drinking water, some municipal water supplies have switched disinfectants from chlorine to chloramine, which minimizes trihalomethane formation.

Mechanism of Toxicity: Chloramine gas decomposes in mucous membranes to form hydrochlorous acid and ammonia. Upon contact with moisture, hydrochlorous acid liberates hydrochloric acid and nascent oxygen, which cause cellular injury and respiratory irritation. The decreased solubility of chloramine compared to chlorine allows less absorption into upper airway mucous membranes and increased delivery to distal airways and alveoli.

Chloramine inhibits various enzyme systems, including carbonic anhydrase, aldehyde dehydrogenase, and superoxide dismutase in vitro; the contribution of enzyme inhibition to toxicity is unknown. Hemolytic anemia is caused by oxidation of erythrocyte hemoglobin to methemoglobin, and inhibition of the hexose monophosphate shunt pathway.

Toxic Dose: Severe cases have involved prolonged exposure to fumes over several hours or days in a closed, poorly ventilated room or house, or brief exposures to very high concentrations in a small space. Most patients with severe pneumonitis ignored initial respiratory irritant symptoms, resulting in delayed treatment.

Signs and Symptoms: Minimal exposure causes immediate eye, nose, and throat irritation, coughing, facial flushing, nausea, and vomiting, which resolve within several hours after termination of exposure. Prolonged or excessive exposure leads to toxic pneumonitis, with symptoms of nonproductive cough, dyspnea, tachypnea, headache, hemoptysis, and tachycardia, which may progress to respiratory failure. Physical examination often shows diffuse rales, rhonchi, and wheezing. A chest roentgenogram in severe cases shows diffuse bilateral interstitial infiltrates, consistent with adult respiratory distress syndrome. Abnormal roentgenographic findings may lag behind pulmonary function abnormalities by several days. Pulsus paradoxicus, caused by high intrapleural pressure, is present in patients with obstructive signs. In severe cases, residual interstitial infiltrates and obstructive defects may persist for 9 months or longer.

Diagnostic Testing: Chloramine is not detected in routine drug screens. Levels are not available or clinically useful.

General Treatment: Treatment is supportive. Administer 100% oxygen as needed for respiratory support. In severe exposures the need for mechanical ventilation should be anticipated.

Decontamination: (Refer to the treatment section p 6 for the appropriate use of these techniques.) Patients should be moved to fresh air immediately and start receiving oxygen, if available, if respiratory symptoms are present.

Antidote: No specific antidotes are available.

Specific Treatment: Supplemental oxygen, bronchodilators, or mechanical ventilation with positive end-expiratory pressure (PEEP) may be required. Patients should be monitored closely for signs of infection and treated promptly. Moderate fluid restriction, with initial fluids at 70% maintenance, is recommended. Additional fluids may be necessary to support cardiovascular function and provide nutritional support.

Patient Monitoring: Pulmonary function may be monitored for the short term with continuous pulse oximetry, chest roentgenograms, and determinations of serial arterial blood gases. Pulmonary function tests should be performed periodically in children with residual signs or symptoms.

Enhanced Elimination: Enhanced elimination techniques are of no proven value.

References

Dunn S, Ozere RL. Ammonia inhalation poisoning—household variety. *Can Med Assoc J.* 1966;94:401

Faigel HC. Hazards to health: mixtures of household cleaning agents. *N Engl J Med.* 1964;271:618

Gapany-Gapanavicius M, Molho M, Tirosh M. Chloramine-induced pneumonitis from mixing household cleaning agents. *Br Med J.* 1982;285:1086

Minami M, Katsumata M, Miyake K, Inagaki H, et al. Dangerous mixture of household detergents in an old-style toilet: a case report with simulation experiments of the working environment and warning of potential hazard relevant to the general environment. *Hum Exp Toxicol.* 1992;11:27-34

Reisz GR, Gammon RS. Toxic pneumonitis from mixing household cleaners. *Chest.* 1986;89:49-52

Chlorine Gas

Available Forms and Sources: Chlorine is a greenish-yellow gas used commercially as a disinfectant and for water purification. It is heavier than air, has a pungent odor, and is generally available as a liquid under pressure. Solid chlorine-releasing products used in residential pools and spas may be a source of exposure in children. Mixing bleach with acids liberates chlorine.

Mechanism of Toxicity: Chlorine is an active oxidizing agent. Injury occurs from the oxidizing effect of nascent oxygen on cell components, free oxygen radical damage, and the caustic effect of hydrochloric acid liberated upon contact of chlorine with water. Pathologic studies demonstrated initial sloughing of airway epithelia followed by an intense inflammatory response, bronchitis, bronchiectasis, and bronchiolitis obliterans. Peribronchial fibrosis may be the mechanism of toxicity in patients with persistently decreased residual volume.

Toxic Dose: Low levels of chlorine gas exposure (1 to 2 ppm) can usually be tolerated for up to 8 hours without undue discomfort. The odor is detected at 3 to 5 ppm, and 1 hour of exposure at this level may cause mild symptoms. At 15 to 30 ppm, exposure causes moderate symptoms, whereas at 40 to 60 ppm the symptoms are severe to life threatening. Exposure to 1000 ppm (0.1%) is rapidly fatal.

Signs and Symptoms: Mild effects include a burning sensation in the mucous membranes of the nose, mouth, and throat, and eye irritation. A slight cough may develop.

Moderate effects include severe irritation of the mucous membranes of the nose, mouth, throat, and eyes often accompanied by a distressing, sometimes paroxysmal cough, which may result in hematemesis. Headache, muscle weakness, wheezing, nausea, nasal-pharyngeal pruritus, hoarseness, chest pain, tachypnea, and palpitations may occur. Anxiety is usually present. A few rales may be heard in the chest; a chest roentgenogram is usually normal.

Severe effects include a productive cough and difficulty breathing. Cyanosis is frequently observed. Rales may be heard throughout the lungs because of edema and congestion. Acute pulmonary effects can include pulmonary edema, bacterial pneumonia, laryngotracheobronchitis, obstructive ventilatory impairment, hypoxemia, metabolic acidosis, and bronchiolitis obliterans. A chest roentgenogram may be normal, but an expirogram may show considerable expiratory reduction. Productive cough, bronchial rales, and an abnormal expirogram may persist for several days. Vomiting may be severe with hematemesis. Death due to progressive respiratory failure has been reported.

A single acute high concentration exposure may produce reactive airways dysfunction syndrome (RADS), a chronic asthma-like illness.

Diagnostic Testing: Chlorine is not detected in a routine drug screen. Levels are not available or clinically useful.

General Treatment: Treatment is supportive. Administer 100% oxygen as needed for respiratory support. In severe exposures the need for mechanical ventilation should be anticipated.

Decontamination: (Refer to the treatment section p 6 for the appropriate use of these techniques.) The victim should be moved to fresh air and 100% oxygen administered if available and respiratory symptoms are present.

Rinse exposed eyes with tepid water. If dermal exposure has occurred, remove clothing and rinse skin thoroughly. If chlorine-generating compounds are ingested, rinse out mouth; do not induce vomiting.

Antidote: No specific antidotes are available.

Specific Treatment: After mild exposure, treatment consists of removing the victim from the source of exposure. In most patients, signs and symptoms clear within a few minutes to an hour.

Following moderate or severe exposures, the patient should lie down with head and shoulders elevated. Administer oxygen in periods of a few minutes at a time until the cough and anxiety are relieved. Nebulized sodium bicarbonate (4 mL of a 3.75% solution) may provide rapid relief of cough, shortness of breath, and tachypnea, but has not been sufficiently studied to recommend its routine use. Bronchoconstriction may be treated with inhaled bronchodilators, subcutaneous epinephrine, or intravenous aminophylline. A sedative-containing cough syrup is useful. Symptoms will abate in most patients within a few hours; however, activity should be restricted for 24 hours to observe the patient for a possible exacerbation of symptoms.

Following patient exposure to a high concentration of chlorine gas, shock, coma, and respiratory arrest may be present. Resuscitation measures, including administration of 100% oxygen and methods to combat shock, may be required. Corticosteroids and/or positive end expiratory pressure (PEEP) may be helpful for pulmonary edema. Moderate fluid restriction, with initial fluids at 70% maintenance, is recommended. Additional fluids may be necessary to support cardiovascular function. Patients should be monitored closely for signs of infection and treated promptly.

Patient Monitoring: Pulmonary function and arterial blood gases should be monitored. Cardiovascular monitoring should be instituted for severe exposures.

Enhanced Elimination: Enhanced elimination techniques are of no proven value.

References

Donnelly SC, FitzGerald MX. Reactive airways dysfunction (RADS) due to chlorine gas exposure. *Irish J Med Sci.* 1990;159:275-276

Fleta J, Calvo C, Zuniga J, Castellano M, Bueno M. Intoxication of 76 children by chlorine gas. *Hum Toxicol.* 1986;5:99-100

Givan DC, Eigen H, Tepper RS. Longitudinal evaluation of pulmonary function in an infant following chlorine gas exposure. *Pediatr Pulmonol.* 1989;6:191-194

Heidemann SM, Goetting MG. Treatment of acute hypoxemic respiratory failure caused by chlorine exposure. *Pediatr Emerg Care.* 1991;7:87-88

Pherwani AV, Khanna SA, Patel RB. Effect of chlorine gas leak on the pulmonary functions of school children. *Indian J Pediatr.* 1989;56:125-128

Schwartz DA, Smith DD, Lakshminarayan S. The pulmonary sequelae associated with accidental inhalation of chlorine gas. *Chest.* 1990;97:820-825

Vinsel PJ. Treatment of acute chlorine gas inhalation with nebulized sodium bicarbonate. *J Emerg Med.* 1990;8:327-329

Cyanide

Available Forms and Sources: Cyanide (CN) is produced by combustion of many substances, including plastics, polyurethane, wool, and silk. Industrial sources include silver and gold extraction, chemical laboratories, and electroplating. Acetonitrile (used in false fingernail solvents and analytical laboratories), propionitrile, and acrylonitrile are metabolized in the liver to CN. Cyanogenic plants or nuts include apricot and peach pits; apple, pear, plum, and cherry seeds; almonds; and bamboo sprouts. Nitroprusside also contains CN groups that are released during its metabolism or reaction with light.

Mechanism of Toxicity: Cyanide inhibits cellular respiration by interfering with oxygen use in the cytochrome oxidase system. Severe tissue hypoxia and metabolic (lactic) acidosis result. Nitriles (eg, acetonitrile) are metabolized by the liver and liberate CN after a delay of 3 to 12 hours.

Toxic Dose: Cyanide gas is rapidly toxic. Many victims of fires in closed spaces die of CN poisoning. Even 5 mL of 20% hydrocyanic acid (HCN) has been fatal when ingested. Cyanide salts (eg, potassium cyanide [KCN]) may produce fatalities in children at 1.2 to 5 mg/kg. Five to ten milliliters of acetonitrile (84%) has produced serious toxic reactions in a child 12 hours after ingestion. An infant died without treatment about 12 hours after ingesting an estimated 15 to 30 mL of acetonitrile. Prolonged nitroprusside infusion in patients with renal compromise or in excessive doses has produced signs of CN toxicity.

   The cyanide content of cyanogenic plants is too variable to estimate a toxic dose. Casual ingestion of a few seeds or pits is very unlikely to cause toxicity.

Signs and Symptoms: Progression and severity of symptoms depend on the dose, route, and duration of exposure. Cyanide gas inhalation can be fatal within minutes with the appearance of skin flushing, hypertension, headache, and hyperpnea, followed rapidly by profound metabolic acidosis, confusion, loss of consciousness, seizures, and respiratory arrest. Cyanosis may be absent or may appear late in the exposure. Venous blood may be bright red, and retinal veins and arteries may appear similarly red. An odor of bitter almonds on the breath may be noted. Cardiac monitoring may show evidence of myocardial ischemia.

Lethal CN ingestions produce a similar but less rapid progression of symptoms. Onset of symptoms can be delayed 3 to 12 hours following acetonitrile ingestion. Nausea and vomiting occur in the first few hours, followed by tachycardia, hypertension, excitation, hyperpnea, and skin flushing, which may progress to lethargy, bradycardia, hypotension, seizures, coma, respiratory arrest, and death. Coingestion of acetone delays onset of CN toxicity from acetonitrile for up to 24 hours.

Nausea, vomiting, metabolic acidosis, headache, dyspnea, ataxia, and confusion characterize nitroprusside toxicity, which can occur after dose escalation in patients with renal impairment or when high-dose infusions are administered longer than 2 to 3 days.

Diagnostic Testing: Cyanide is not detected in a routine drug screen. A whole blood or plasma CN determination can be diagnostic, but is not routinely available, and the assay may require 6 hours or longer to perform. Because CN is an intracellular toxin, blood or plasma CN levels may not correlate with symptoms. A serum thiocyanate (a cyanide metabolite) determination is more widely available but is less useful to confirm CN toxicity or determine the severity of intoxication. Thiocyanate levels may be elevated during nitroprusside therapy.

The pO_2 may be normal on an arterial blood gas, despite respiratory distress. A markedly diminished pO_2 or saturation difference between arterial and venous blood suggests either CN or hydrogen sulfide poisoning.

General Treatment: Because significant symptoms are possible, the need for life support measures including intubation and ventilation with 100% oxygen should be anticipated. Oxygen (100%) should be administered if CN gas is suspected (such as in a fire in a closed space).

Decontamination: (Refer to the treatment section p 6 for the appropriate use of these techniques.) Emesis is not recommended because the onset of CN toxicity after oral ingestion of HCN or KCN is too rapid, and significant absorption of liquid nitriles may occur before emesis is induced. Gastric lavage and activated charcoal may reduce the absorption of liquid CN compounds or nitriles.

Antidote: The Lilly cyanide antidote kit contains three agents administered in the following order: (1) an amyl nitrite crushable ampule (crushed and inhaled for 30 seconds while the other agents are being prepared); (2) sodium nitrite for intravenous use (0.33 mL/kg initially); and (3) sodium thiosulfate for intravenous use (1.65 mL/kg of the 25% solution up to a maximum of 50 mL). Methemoglobin levels should be monitored and should not exceed 20% to 30% (70% is fatal). The nitrites produce methemoglobin to which CN binds, thus freeing tissue cytochrome oxidase to resume cellular respiration. Thiosulfate acts as a sulfhydryl donor to increase the activity of rhodanese, the rate-limiting enzyme in CN detoxification. This enzyme converts CN to thiocyanate, which is then excreted in urine. Nitrites are vasodilators and may cause hypotension, headaches, vomiting, or fainting.

Because methemoglobin does not transport oxygen, therapy with nitrites may be omitted in patients likely to already have high methemoglobin levels or in patients with mixed CN and carbon monoxide exposure (such as in a fire in a closed space), cyanotic patients, or those with severe cardiovascular disease who may not tolerate hypotension. Sodium thiosulfate alone, without prior nitrite administration, may be an effective antidote. Hyperbaric oxygen therapy has been recommended for victims of CN gas exposure and closed-space fires but timely transport may not be feasible. Hydroxocobalamin (vitamin B_{12a}) is an experimental antidote that binds to CN to form cyanocobalamin (vitamin B_{12}), which is renally excreted; unfortunately, current clinical trials do not include children. Commercially available hydroxocobalamin is too dilute and packaged in quantities that are too small to be usable for this purpose.

Specific Treatment: Sodium bicarbonate and electrolyte solutions should be administered to correct metabolic acidosis and restore normal electrolyte balance. Intravenous or intraosseous fluid administration may be necessary shortly after exposure.

Patient Monitoring: Monitor vital signs, mental status, blood gases, and electrolyte levels.

Enhanced Elimination: Enhanced elimination techniques are of no proven value.

References

Boggild MD, Peck RW, Tomson CRV. Acetonitrile ingestion: delayed onset of cyanide poisoning due to concurrent ingestion of acetone. *Postgrad Med J.* 1990;66:40-41

Caravati EM, Litovitz TL. Pediatric cyanide intoxication and death from an acetonitrile-containing cosmetic. *JAMA.* 1988;260:3470-3473

Hall AH, Kulig KW, Rumack BH. Suspected cyanide poisoning in smoke inhalation: complications of sodium nitrite therapy. *J Toxicol Clin.* 1989;9:3-9

Johnson WS, Hall AH, Rumack BH. Cyanide poisoning successfully treated without therapeutic methemoglobin levels. *Am J Emerg Med.* 1989;7:437-440

Losek JD, Rock AL, Boldt RR. Cyanide poisoning from a cosmetic nail remover. *Pediatrics.* 1991;88:337-340

Michaelis HC, Clemens C, Kijewski H, Neurath H, Eggert A. Acetonitrile serum concentrations and cyanide blood levels in a case of suicidal oral acetonitrile ingestion. *J Toxicol Clin Toxicol.* 1991;29:447-458

Way JL. Cyanide intoxication and its mechanism of antagonism. *Ann Rev Pharmacol Toxicol.* 1984;24:451-481

Cyanoacrylate Adhesives

Available Forms and Sources: These products are rapid-bonding, high-strength adhesives, frequently referred to as "super glue." They are sold in small tubes and in small dropper bottles.

Mechanism of Toxicity: Cyanoacrylate adhesives bond instantly to soft tissues and produce a firm bond. Primary irritation occurs when bonded surfaces are mechanically pulled apart, and when small pieces of polymerized material produce a rough surface. Corneal abrasions are frequently noted following ocular contact with cyanoacrylate adhesives. The vapors of cyanoacrylate adhesives may be irritating, particularly after heating. Cyanide gas is not released unless combustion occurs.

Toxic Dose: Toxicity following dermal or ocular contact is a result of adhesion and mechanical irritation, and is not dose related.

Signs and Symptoms: If these adhesives are ingested, significant symptoms are not anticipated.

Ocular exposure. Cyanoacrylate adhesives rapidly bond eyelids together. These agents may also cause corneal abrasions, keratoconjunctivitis, or both, largely by mechanical irritation. Permanent ocular damage is rare.

Inhalation. Cyanoacrylate adhesive vapors may be irritating, particularly after they are heated. Bronchospasm and allergic rhinitis may occur in sensitive individuals. Panic attacks have been reported following inhalation.

Diagnostic Testing: Cyanoacrylates are not detected in routine drug screens.

General Treatment: Significant acute symptoms are not expected.

Decontamination: (Refer to the treatment section p 6 for the appropriate use of these techniques.) Treatment of dermal exposures addresses measures to release the adhesive bond, where needed. Untreated, bonded surfaces separate in a few days. Prolonged soaking in warm, soapy water or the application of acetone may promote separation. Mineral oil, vegetable oil, or petroleum jelly applied over a period of time may aid in softening the adhesive bond and removing the adherent glue. The latter agents are particularly suitable for sensitive areas of skin and near the eyes. Specific solvents are marketed to dissolve cyanoacrylate adhesive bonds, but may pose inherent toxic hazards themselves and should be used cautiously in keeping with the manufacturer's instructions. Surgical separation of tissues is generally unnecessary.

Ocular exposures should be evaluated for corneal abrasions and retained bits of glue under the lids. If the lids are bonded together, use of mineral oil soaks, petroleum jelly applied to the adhered area, or both may assist in dissolving the bond. Irrigation of the conjunctival area should be carried out to the extent possible. Surgical separation of bonded eyelids is occasionally appropriate when pain from retained debris is present or when dissolution of the bonded surfaces cannot be accomplished over several days by other means.

Antidote: No specific antidotes are available or necessary.

Specific Treatment: Corneal abrasions should be treated with antibiotics, patching, and appropriate follow-up. Bronchospasm can be treated with bronchodilators and antiinflammatory agents, as necessary.

Enhanced Elimination: Enhanced elimination techniques are of no proven value.

References

Bock GW. Skin exposure to cyanoacrylate adhesive. *Ann Emerg Med.* 1984;13:486

Dean BS, Krenzelok EP. Cyanoacrylates and corneal abrasion. *Clin Toxicol.* 1989;27:169-172

Kopp SK, McKay RT, Moller DR, Cassedy K, Brooks SM. Asthma and rhinitis due to ethylcyanoacrylate instant glue. *Ann Intern Med.* 1985;102:613

Yeragani VK, Pohl R, Balon R. Panic attacks and exposure to chemical agents. *Am J Psychiatry.* 1988;145:532

Ethylene Glycol

Available Forms and Sources: Ethylene glycol is a liquid used as an automotive antifreeze. It may also be present in windshield deicers and brake fluid. It is colorless, with a faint odor and a sweet taste. Because products differ greatly in their ingredients, a regional poison center should be contacted for specific product information.

Mechanism of Toxicity: Ethylene glycol is metabolized by hepatic enzymes to glycolaldehyde, glyoxylic acid, oxalic acid, and formic acid. Both the parent compound and metabolites produce toxicity. After a delay of up to 12 to 24 hours, oxalate crystals may appear in urine and be deposited in tissues, causing acute renal failure and cardiac and central nervous system toxicity.

Toxic Dose: An adult fatality has been reported following an ingestion of 100 mL (about 1.4 mL/kg) of 100% ethylene glycol. Patients have survived when higher doses have been ingested and prompt, appropriate therapy was instituted. The toxic dose in children is not established.

Signs and Symptoms: Ethylene glycol produces central nervous system depression, and its metabolites cause metabolic (anion gap) acidosis, hypocalcemia, further central nervous system depression, and tissue damage. Three clinical stages of poisoning have been described. Progression and severity of signs in these stages depend on the dose ingested. Stage 1 (from 1 to 12 hours after ingestion) is characterized by nausea, vomiting, metabolic acidosis, and progressive central nervous system signs including elation, nystagmus, myoclonic jerks, coma, and convulsions. The patient may appear inebriated but lack the characteristic odor of alcohol. Laboratory assessment reveals a low level of serum bicarbonate and a low pH, an increased anion gap, and an osmolal gap (see p 28 for calculations). Stage 2 occurs 12 to 24 hours after exposure. Signs of this stage are primarily cardiovascular including tachycardia, tachypnea, mild hypertension, congestive heart failure, and circulatory collapse. Hypocalcemia exacerbates cardiac toxic effects. Skeletal muscle pain with elevated levels of serum creatine phosphokinase has been reported. Patients in stage 3 (24 to 72 hours after exposure) show renal involvement, including flank pain, oliguria, acute tubular necrosis, and renal failure. Acute tubular necrosis has been reported as early as 12 hours after ingestion.

Diagnostic Testing: Ethylene glycol is not detected by most routine drug screens. A serum ethylene glycol level is diagnostic but may not be readily available. Results may require hours to days depending on the availability of the reference laboratory. Analysis by gas chromatography may give false-positive results for ethylene glycol in the presence of propylene glycol (a vehicle in some parenteral medications) or some inborn errors of metabolism (such as methylmalonic acidemia). The severity of acidosis (ie, the serum bicarbonate level) is better correlated with clinical severity than is the ethylene glycol level.

If ethylene glycol levels are not readily available, a freezing point depression osmolality can be used to estimate the osmolal gap (see p 28), which can be used to estimate the ethylene glycol level, as shown:

$$\begin{matrix} \text{ESTIMATED} \\ \text{BLOOD} \\ \text{LEVEL} \\ \text{(mg/dL, or mg\%)} \end{matrix} = \text{OSMOLAL GAP x 6.2}$$

Metabolites of ethylene glycol contribute to the osmolal gap and can result in overestimation of the blood level. Also, estimation of blood levels of ethylene glycol by this method is not reliable if an alcohol (ie, ethanol, methanol) was also ingested in significant amounts.

Antifreeze usually contains fluorescein, which is rapidly excreted in urine. Fluorescence of the urine under ultraviolet light (Wood's lamp) may confirm antifreeze ingestion in questionable cases, but the absence of fluorescence does not rule out ingestion.

General Treatment: Significant acute symptoms are not expected. The need for life support measures including respiratory support and seizure treatment should be anticipated. Ethanol infusion and dialysis may be necessary.

Decontamination: (Refer to the treatment section p 6 for the appropriate use of these techniques.) In general, emesis should not be attempted because of the risk of central nervous system depression. Gastric lavage is likely to be most useful within 30 to 60 minutes after ingestion, since ethylene glycol is rapidly and completely absorbed from the gastrointestinal tract within 1 to 4 hours. Gastric lavage may be helpful several hours after ingestion of massive amounts or if gastric motility is slowed by another ingestant, food, or coma. Activated charcoal does not bind ethylene glycol.

Antidote: (See Table 2, p 16, for specific dosing.) Ethanol is the preferred substrate for alcohol dehydrogenase and blocks ethylene glycol metabolism and the formation of toxic metabolites. A loading dose of ethanol should be given when there are clinical signs and a history of ethylene glycol ingestion, severe or persistent metabolic acidosis, or a blood ethylene glycol level of 25 mg/dL or higher. Ethanol loading is also recommended in symptomatic patients who are awaiting hemodialysis or the results of ethylene glycol determinations. After ethanol loading, repeated dosing (oral or nasogastric) or a continuous intravenous infusion of ethanol should be started. Oral ethanol may cause nausea or emesis. Intravenous infusion is the most reliable route of administration, but phlebitis may occur, and many hospitals may not stock intravenous ethanol. Blood ethanol levels should be monitored and the dose adjusted to maintain a blood ethanol level of 100 to 150 mg/dL. Ethanol administration increases the elimination half-life of ethylene glycol to about 17 hours.

Pyridoxine and thiamine serve as cofactors in the metabolism of ethylene glycol and may be administered following significant ingestions (see Table 2, p 16, for specific dosing).

4-Methylpyrazole is an experimental agent that inhibits alcohol dehydrogenase, thus inhibiting ethylene glycol metabolism. It is not commercially available.

Specific Treatment: Acidosis may require large doses of intravenous sodium bicarbonate. Treat hypocalcemia with intravenous calcium chloride, administered slowly. Administer intravenous fluids to maintain adequate urine flow, but do not use diuretics (eg, furosemide, mannitol) if oxalate crystals are present in the urine of an oliguric patient.

Patient Monitoring: Obtain values for serum electrolytes, serum urea nitrogen, glucose, and freezing point depression osmolality to calculate osmolal and anion gaps. Urinary oxalate crystals and metabolic acidosis may be delayed for several hours after ingestion. Monitor urine output, specific gravity, proteinuria, and microscopic crystalluria.

Enhanced Elimination: Ethylene glycol is rapidly removed by hemodialysis. Indications for hemodialysis include progressive deterioration of vital signs, refractory metabolic acidosis, massive oxalate crystalluria, renal failure, or an ethylene glycol level of 50 mg/dL or higher. Ethanol infusion should be continued during hemodialysis and requires an increase in the ethanol dose to maintain a blood ethanol level of 100 to 150 mg/dL.

References

Baud FJ, Galliot M, Astier A, Vu Bien D, et al. Treatment of ethylene glycol poisoning with intravenous 4-methylpyrazole. *N Engl J Med.* 1988; 319:97-100

Burkhart KK, Kulig KW. The other alcohols: methanol, ethylene glycol, and isopropanol. *Emerg Med Clin North Am.* 1990;8:913-928

Litovitz T. The alcohols: ethanol, methanol, isopropanol, ethylene glycol. *Pediatr Clin North Am.* 1986;33:311-323

Saladino R, Shannon M. Accidental and intentional poisonings with ethylene glycol in infancy: diagnostic clues and management. *Pediatr Emerg Care.* 1991;7:93-96

Shoemaker JD, Lynch RE, Hoffmann JW, Sly WS. Misidentification of propionic acid as ethylene glycol in a patient with methylmalonic acidemia. *J Pediatr.* 1992;120:417-421

Winter ML, Ellis MD, Snodgrass WR. Urine fluorescence using a Wood's lamp to detect the antifreeze additive sodium fluorescein: a qualitative adjunctive test in suspected ethylene glycol ingestions. *Ann Emerg Med.* 1990;19:663-667

Woolf AD, Wynshaw Boris A, Rinaldo P, Levy HL. Intentional infantile ethylene glycol poisoning presenting as an inherited metabolic disorder. *J Pediatr.* 1992;120:421-424

Herbicides - Chlorophenoxy

Available Forms and Sources: Commonly available chlorophenoxy herbicides include 2,4-dichlorophenoxyacetic acid (2,4-D), 2,4,5-trichlorophenoxypropionic acid (Silvex), and 4-chloro-2-methylphenoxyacetic acid (MCPA). The compound 2,4,5-T (2,4,5-trichlorophenoxyacetic acid) is no longer marketed in the United States.

Mechanism of Toxicity: These agents dissociate in water into strong acids. A weak inhibitor of oxidative phosphorylation, 2,4-D also injures striated muscle and may be toxic to peripheral nerve tissue.

Toxic Dose: In adults, clinical toxicity has been reported after an intravenous dose of 3600 mg, and a death occurred after an ingestion of 6000 mg (80 mg/kg). An adult who ingested 500 mg/d for 21 days had no clinical effects noted. Gastrointestinal decontamination has been suggested following an ingested dose exceeding 40 mg/kg. In one study 6% of an applied forearm dose was absorbed.

Signs and Symptoms: After large exposures, weakness, coma, hyperthermia, metabolic acidosis, myalgia, and myoglobinuria have been noted, as well as signs of irritation of the skin, eyes, respiratory tract, and gastrointestinal tract. These agents also appear to be mild hepatotoxins and nephrotoxins.

Diagnostic Testing: These compounds are not detected in a routine drug screen. Chlorophenoxy herbicide levels can be obtained, but are unlikely to be clinically useful.

General Treatment: Significant acute symptoms are not anticipated.

Decontamination: (Refer to the treatment section p 6 for the appropriate use of these techniques.) Emesis can be used if instituted early. Gastric lavage can also be used. Administration of activated charcoal may be preferable with substantial ingestions. Ocular exposures should be treated with thorough water flushing. Dermal exposures should be thoroughly decontaminated with water and a weak detergent solution.

Antidote: No specific antidotes are available.

Specific Treatment: Treatment is supportive. There is no specific treatment.

Patient Monitoring: After substantial exposures, levels of serum electrolytes, serum creatinine, and hepatic enzymes should be monitored. Urinalysis should be performed, including evaluation for the possibility of myoglobinuria.

Enhanced Elimination: Alkaline diuresis improves the elimination of 2,4-D and prevents renal injury from myoglobinuria. It
should be reserved for substantial or symptomatic exposures.·

References

Mortensen ML. Management of acute childhood poisonings caused
by selected insecticides and herbicides. *Pediatr Clin North Am.* 1986;33:
421-445

Wells WD, Wright N, Yeoman WB. Clinical features and management of
poisoning with 2,4-D and mecoprop. *Clin Toxicol.* 1981;18:273-276

Hydrocarbons
(Including Volatile Solvents)

Available Forms and Sources: Aliphatic and aromatic
hydrocarbons including propane, butane, isobutane, hexane,
heptane, octane, benzene, toluene, and xylene are common constituents of fuels such as kerosene and gasoline. These compounds also are commonly found in glues, propellants, lighter
fluids, inks, paints, pesticides, furniture polishes, and paint
thinners. Abuse of these agents by inhalation is common (see
inhalants, p 152).

Halogenated hydrocarbons include methylene chloride,
chloroform, carbon tetrachloride, 1,1,1-trichloroethane, trichloroethylene, freons, perchloroethylene, and many others. These
hydrocarbons are found in propellants, degreasing solvents, dry
cleaning solutions, and computer keyboard cleaners.

Mechanism of Toxicity: Most deaths following ingestion of
petroleum distillates result from aspiration into the lung. Products
with low viscosity (30 to 60 SSU) such as lighter fluids pose a
high aspiration hazard because of their tendency to spread over a
large surface area. Chemical pneumonitis results from aspiration
of as little as a few milliliters of the product. Aspiration usually
occurs at the time of ingestion or upon emesis. Large amounts of
most hydrocarbons can be tolerated by ingestion if the product is
not aspirated.

All of these materials are lipophilic, which leads to defatting of the skin and mucous membranes, resulting in irritation and, with prolonged exposure, chemical burns. Once absorbed from the skin, gastrointestinal tract, or lung, these compounds accumulate in brain lipids, causing central nervous system depression. Sensitization of the myocardium may lead to dysrhythmias and sudden death. Metabolites of some of these compounds are hepatic and renal toxins.

Benzene is a known human carcinogen. Several chlorinated solvents are possible human carcinogens.

Toxic Dose: The toxic dose depends on the specific compound and the route of exposure. Petroleum products with high viscosity, such as grease, have limited toxic potential. Low-viscosity products, such a mineral seal oil, have a high aspiration potential.

Signs and Symptoms: Dermal, ocular, and aural exposures lead to erythema and irritation. Blisters and sloughing of the skin may occur.

Acute inhalation symptoms may include the rapid development of intoxication accompanied by euphoria, disinhibition, and the feeling of invulnerability. Dysphoric symptoms occur with higher doses and may include hallucinations, agitation, and confusion. Central nervous system depression including unconsciousness and respiratory depression may ensue. Convulsions are uncommon but have been reported.

Chronic inhalation exposure leads to the gradual onset of serious and, in part, irreversible central nervous system injury. (see inhalants, p 152).

Ingestion of solvents frequently leads to immediate gagging with pulmonary aspiration. Significant aspiration may lead to the rapid development of severe chemical pneumonitis with respiratory failure requiring mechanical ventilation. Aspiration is frequently accompanied by the rapid development of low-grade fever. Ingestion also produces significant gastric irritation with the risk of vomiting and further aspiration.

Absorption of significant quantities of solvents through the lung, skin, or gastrointestinal tract can produce other systemic symptoms, including cardiac dysrhythmias, that may cause sudden death and occasionally liver and renal abnormalities.

Diagnostic Testing: Routine toxicology screening does not identify these agents, although special techniques can be used to identify some substances in blood or exhaled air. Urine may be analyzed for metabolites of xylene, toluene, or trichloroethylene. Routine chest roentgenograms are not necessary or useful unless respiratory symptoms are present.

General Treatment: Because significant symptoms are possible, the need for life support measures including respiratory and cardiovascular support should be anticipated.

Decontamination: (Refer to the treatment section p 6 for the appropriate use of these techniques.) Solvents on the skin should be removed with large volumes of soap and water. Eyes should be copiously rinsed with water or saline for at least 10 to 15 minutes. Inhalation exposures usually respond to moving the person to fresh air. If the person loses consciousness, supplemental oxygen may be necessary.

The ingestion of simple hydrocarbons such as kerosene or gasoline usually does not require decontamination. Because the primary problem associated with these agents is aspiration pneumonia, emesis should not be induced, nor should nasogastric or orogastric tubes be inserted. Activated charcoal is not effective at binding most of these agents and should not be administered. Removal of the solvent from the stomach may be necessary because it possesses inherent toxicity (benzene) or is a vehicle for a more toxic agent (pesticides). In these situations emesis can be performed under controlled conditions in the emergency department. Gastric lavage can also be used, although it is recommended that a cuffed endotracheal tube be inserted before the lavage tube.

Antidote: No specific antidotes are available.

Specific Treatment: There are no systematic data assessing the effectiveness of various treatments for hydrocarbon aspiration pneumonitis. Corticosteroids are frequently recommended but are of no proven value. Anecdotal reports indicate possible value from the use of surfactant replacement products. Extracorporeal membrane oxygenation (ECMO) has been used successfully in a few patients with life-threatening respiratory failure. Generally, aggressive supportive respiratory care is the standard treatment modality.

Patient Monitoring: Monitor arterial blood gases and sequential chest roentgenograms in patients with respiratory symptoms.

Enhanced Elimination: Enhanced elimination techniques are of no proven value.

References

Bass M. Sudden sniffing death. *JAMA.* 1970;212:2075-2079

Flanagan RJ, Ruprah TJ, Meredith TJ, Ramsey JD. An introduction to the clinical toxicology of volatile substances. *Drug Saf.* 1990;5:359-383

Klein BL, Simon JE. Hydrocarbon poisoning. *Pediatr Clin North Am.* 1986;33:411-419.

Machado B, Cross K, Snodgrass WR. Accidental hydrocarbon ingestion cases telephoned to a regional poison center. *Ann Emerg Med.* 1988;17:804-807

Meredith TJ, Ruprah M, Liddle A, Flanagan RJ. Diagnosis and treatment of acute poisoning with volatile substances. *Hum Toxicol.* 1989;8:277-286

Wason S, Gibler WB, Hassan M. Ventricular tachycardia associated with non-freon aerosol propellants. *JAMA.* 1986;256:78-80

Hydrogen Sulfide

Available Forms and Sources: Hydrogen sulfide is a naturally occurring colorless gas. It is heavier than air and has a characteristic odor of rotten eggs. Common sources are oil and gas wells, livestock wastes, and organic sewage that has reacted with bacteria or acids. It is also a by-product of a number of industrial processes.

Mechanism of Toxicity: Hydrogen sulfide inhibits cytochrome oxidase, leading to tissue hypoxia and diffuse cellular dysfunction. Severe metabolic acidosis results from the conversion to anaerobic metabolism. At very low concentrations (10 to 50 ppm) hydrogen sulfide is an irritant to the eyes and lungs.

Toxic Dose: Exposure to levels of more than 0.1% (1000 ppm) causes death within minutes. Concentrations in the range of 10 to 100 ppm (0.001% to 0.01%) are unpleasant because of the odor and produce symptoms of irritation but are not life-threatening. The odor of hydrogen sulfide is detectable at about 0.02 ppm but is no longer detectable above 100 ppm due to olfactory saturation; toxic concentrations, therefore, are not discernible by smell.

Signs and Symptoms: Irritation of the eyes and respiratory tract generally appear before systemic symptoms.

At toxic concentrations, the primary target organ is the central nervous system. Progressive signs and symptoms include headache, weakness, vertigo, nystagmus, nausea and vomiting, dyspnea, pulmonary edema, coma, and seizures. Cardiac dysrhythmias and cardiogenic shock may occur.

Diagnostic Testing: The diagnosis generally is made by history or detection of the odor. There is no readily available diagnostic test. Hydrogen sulfide is not detected in a drug screen.

General Treatment: Treatment is supportive with the use of 100% oxygen delivered by a non-rebreather mask or endotracheal tube.

Decontamination: (Refer to the treatment section p 6 for the appropriate use of these techniques.) Because exposure is almost always by inhalation, the patient should be moved to fresh air and oxygen should be administered as soon as possible. Skin, eye, and gastrointestinal decontamination are not generally required.

Antidote: Nitrite-induced methemoglobinemia may be helpful if instituted early. Sulfide reacts with methemoglobin to form sulfhemaglobin, which is rapidly metabolized in the body regenerating hemoglobin. Because the body rapidly metabolizes sulfide even in the absence of methemoglobin, inducing methemoglobinemia is unlikely to be clinically helpful unless it is done within the first few minutes after exposure. Dosing of nitrites should follow the guidelines in the product literature with the Lilly Cyanide Antidote Kit **(see Table 2, p 16, for specific dosing)**. It is not necessary to use the sodium thiosulfate in the kit. Methylene blue should be readily available to reverse excessive methemoglobinemia. The administration of hyperbaric oxygen (3 atm) has been reported to be effective in a few cases.

Specific Treatment: Treatment is supportive. There is no specific treatment.

Patient Monitoring: Monitor methemoglobin levels if nitrites are used as well as arterial blood gases.

Enhanced Elimination: Enhanced elimination techniques are of no proven value.

References

Beauchamp RO Jr, Bus JS, Popp JA, Boreiko CJ, Andjelkovich DA. A critical review of the literature on hydrogen sulfide toxicity. *Crit Rev Toxicol.* 1984;13:25-97

Morse DL, Woodbury MA, Rentmeester K, Farmer D. Death caused by fermenting manure. *JAMA.* 1981;244:63-64

Ravizza AG, Carugo D, Cerchiari EL, Cantadore R, Bianchi GE. The treatment of hydrogen sulfide intoxication: oxygen versus nitrites. *Vet Hum Toxicol.* 1982;24:241-242

Whitcraft DD, Bailey TD, Hart GB. Hydrogen sulfide poisoning treated with hyperbaric oxygen. *J Emerg Med.* 1985;3:23-25

Insecticides - Organophosphate and Carbamate

Available Forms and Sources:

Organophosphate insecticides. Numerous agents in this class are available and may be generally divided into "highly toxic" and "moderately toxic" groups on the basis of toxicity in animals. Some of the most common agents are chlorpyrifos, diazinon, and malathion (all moderately toxic).

Carbamate insecticides. Agents in this class may be similarly grouped into highly toxic and moderately toxic categories. Common substances include aldicarb (highly toxic), propoxur, and carbaryl (both moderately toxic).

Mechanism of Toxicity: These compounds interfere with the normal degradation by cholinesterases of acetylcholine (and similar esters), thus "jamming" transmission of impulses in muscarinic and nicotinic nerve fibers. Affected enzymes include acetylcholinesterase (principally present in red blood cells and neurons), pseudocholinesterase (principally found in serum, hepatocytes, and other organs), and neurotoxic esterase (found in the central nervous system).

Organophosphate compounds interfere noncompetitively with the degradation of acetylcholine (and similar esters). Initially their activity is reversible. For many of the organophosphates, "aging" of the bond between the organophosphate and the active site of the enzyme occurs, rendering the bond permanent and the blockade of enzyme activity irreversible. This aging occurs over the 48 hours following exposure. The specific chemical compound and the host determine the duration of time to permanent interference. Once enzyme activity is permanently abolished, it can be restored only upon synthesis of new enzyme, a process typically requiring weeks to months. Although carbamates also bind to cholinesterase, this bond is reversible over a period of hours.

Toxic Dose: The toxic dose is variable, depending on the concentration and duration of exposure and the amount of enzyme present in the individual and its level of activity. About 3% of otherwise normal individuals have genetically determined low levels of enzyme activity. These products are readily absorbed through the skin and significant toxic effects can occur by this route of exposure.

Signs and Symptoms: Characteristic signs and symptoms include headache, nausea, dizziness, anxiety, and restlessness, progressing to muscle fasciculations, weakness, abdominal cramps, and general exocrine gland hypersecretion. Pulmonary edema may develop and may progress to frank respiratory failure.

Hypersecretion is frequently referred to by the acronym SLUDGE, which stands for *s*alivation, *l*acrimation, *u*rination, *d*efecation, *g*astrointestinal cramps, and *e*mesis. Pupillary constriction is frequently noted, but may be offset by other metabolic effects of the poisoning. Bradycardia or tachycardia may occur, but are not predictable findings. Recurrent weakness caused by a motor polyneuropathy, principally distal, has been reported following exposure to some of these agents, particularly those that "age" neurotoxic esterase. Long-lasting neurobehavioral changes have been reported in adults following large, acute exposures to certain organophosphates. Onset of symptoms may be delayed with some of these compounds, particularly those containing a "thione" group and with dermal exposures.

Diagnostic Testing: These agents are not routinely identified in a drug screen. Detection of organophosphates and carbamates in the blood is made difficult by rapid metabolism. Detection of metabolites in the urine may be possible up to 48 hours after exposure, depending on individual kinetics and the extent of exposure.

Cholinesterase activity may be measured in serum or red blood cells. Serum cholinesterase ("pseudocholinesterase") measurements generally reflect recent exposure over the past several days to weeks. Red blood cell cholinesterase ("RBC acetylcholinesterase") activity, on the other hand, may continue to fall for several days after a single acute exposure and then remain depressed for 1 to 3 months. Enzyme activity may be depressed by other factors, including malnutrition, liver dysfunction, pregnancy, oral contraceptives, and hemolytic anemias.

General Treatment: Because significant symptoms are possible, the need for life support measures including respiratory support and seizure treatment should be anticipated.

Decontamination: **(Refer to the treatment section p 6 for the appropriate use of these techniques.)** Remove as much toxin from the person as possible by removing contaminated clothes and washing exposed surfaces several times with soap and water or a weak detergent solution. Emergency personnel should wear protective clothing while decontaminating patients because these agents are well absorbed through the skin. Leather goods cannot be decontaminated and must be disposed of. Emesis is contraindicated; gastric lavage or activated charcoal treatment should be considered if a potentially toxic dose has been ingested.

Antidote: Atropine antagonizes the muscarinic (SLUDGE) effects of these agents. A test dose of 0.02 mg/kg up to a 1-mg total dose may be administered. Failure to reverse the SLUDGE effects supports a diagnosis of cholinergic poisoning; in the absence of cholinergic excess, such a dose of atropine should dry secretions, increase the heart rate, and dilate the pupils.

If a test dose of atropine confirms cholinergic excess, a sufficient amount of atropine should be administered to restore physiologic equilibrium. Large doses, sometimes even by continuous infusion, are frequently necessary, and may be required for periods of days to weeks. In this situation, a concentrated solution of atropine can be prepared from atropine powder. The end points for atropine therapy are tachycardia (a heart rate of more than 120 beats per minute), diminished secretions, and resolution of pulmonary edema. Pupil size is not a valid indication of adequate atropinization. Atropine may not be effective at reversing respiratory muscle weakness.

If an organophosphate is implicated as the cause of the cholinergic excess, treatment with pralidoxime (2-PAM, Protopam) is generally indicated **(see Table 2, p 16, for specific dosing)** in addition to atropine therapy. Pralidoxime restores some enzyme function before aging has occurred and may ameliorate nicotinic effects including respiratory muscle weakness. Pralidoxime may not reverse central nervous system effects. It is generally not indicated for carbamate poisoning.

Specific Treatment: Usual supportive measures should be followed. Treat respiratory insufficiency with intubation, oxygen, and PEEP. Pulmonary edema may respond to cautious use of diuretics. Seizures may respond to standard anticonvulsant agents or atropine or pralidoxime. Treat cardiac dysrhythmias with standard agents **(see Table 3, p 22, for specific dosing)**.

Patient Monitoring: For symptomatic patients, cardiorespiratory monitoring including arterial blood gases is essential. Fluid status and electrolyte levels should also be closely monitored.

Enhanced Elimination: Enhanced elimination techniques are of no proven value to remove the chemical.

References

Morgan DP. *Recognition and Management of Pesticide Poisonings*. 4th ed. Washington, DC: US Environmental Protection Agency; 1989

Mortensen ML. Management of acute childhood poisonings caused by selected insecticides and herbicides. *Pediatr Clin North Am.* 1986;33:421-445

Rosenstock L, Keifer M, Daniell WE, McConnell R, Claypoole K. Chronic central nervous system effects of acute organophosphate pesticide intoxication. *Lancet.* 1991;338:223-227

Sofer S, Tal A, Shahak E. Carbamate and organophosphate poisoning in early childhood. *Pediatr Emerg Care.* 1989;81:121-126

Thompson DF, Thompson GD, Greenwood RB, Trammel HL. Therapeutic dosing of pralidoxime chloride. *Drug Intell Clin Pharm.* 1987;21:590-593

Zwiener RJ, Ginsburg CM. Organophosphate and carbamate poisoning in infants and children *Pediatrics.* 1988;81:121-126

Isopropyl Alcohol

Available Forms and Sources: Isopropyl alcohol (isopropanol) is a component of solvents, antifreeze, deicing solutions, window cleaners, aftershave lotions, and rubbing alcohol. A clear, colorless liquid found principally in rubbing solutions in various concentrations, it is usually sold in pint bottles with coloration added. It is also used in small concentrations as a solvent in some skin lotions and topical medications.

Mechanism of Toxicity: Isopropanol is metabolized to acetone, both of which are potent central nervous system depressants. They may also cause myocardial depression and peripheral vasodilation, leading to shock. Hypoglycemia with subsequent seizures may occur because the utilization of NAD during the hepatic metabolism of isopropanol causes a decrease in gluconeogenesis.

Toxic Dose: A dose of 1 mL/kg of 70% isopropyl alcohol produces a serum level of 70 mg/dL. Treatment is indicated if more than 0.5 to 1 mL/kg is ingested. Toxic reactions may also occur from inhalation of high concentrations of isopropyl alcohol. Coma has been reported after a child was sponged with rubbing alcohol while being treated for fever.

Signs and Symptoms: Central nervous system depressant effects are about twice those of ethyl alcohol at comparable blood levels. Acute signs and symptoms may develop within 30 minutes after ingestion and include dizziness, headache, incoordination, stupor, or coma. Isopropyl alcohol is irritating to the gastrointestinal tract and is likely to cause vomiting, hematemesis, and diarrhea. Patients may experience hypothermia, bradycardia, hypotension, and even circulatory collapse. Symptoms may persist longer than those associated with ethanol poisoning. Acetonuria, ketosis, and anuria may occur. Pulmonary injury with edema may occur as a result of excretion of the alcohol through the lungs. Myopathy and hemolytic anemias are occasionally seen. Hypoglycemia occurs, particularly in young children.

Diagnostic Testing: Isopropyl alcohol is detected in most routine drug screens. Serum levels may be obtained and are useful in evaluating the exposure. Serum levels greater than 50 to 100 mg/dL indicate the need for close observation of the patient. Isopropyl alcohol concentrations of 50 to 100 mg/dL produce lethargy, 150 to 200 mg/dL induce coma, and levels greater than 400 mg/dL are potentially fatal.

An increased osmolal gap (1 mOsm for each 5.9 mg/dL of isopropyl alcohol and 1 mOsm for each 5.5 mg/dL of acetone), associated with an increased level of serum acetone, a normal blood pH, a decreased serum bicarbonate level, and a normal anion gap, is characteristic of isopropyl alcohol intoxication.

General Treatment: Because significant symptoms are possible, the need for life support measures including respiratory support should be anticipated following large ingestions.

Decontamination: (Refer to the treatment section p 6 for the appropriate use of these techniques.) Emesis is generally not indicated because of the potential for central nervous system depression. Gastric lavage may be useful if instituted within 1 hour of the ingestion of a large quantity of material. Activated charcoal does not bind isopropyl alcohol.

Antidote: No specific antidotes are available.

Specific Treatment: Provide aggressive supportive care as signs and symptoms warrant. If the patient is hypoglycemic, glucose should be administered intravenously.

Patient Monitoring: Monitor serum pH and levels of isopropyl alcohol, acetone, glucose, and serum electrolytes.

Enhanced Elimination: Forced fluid diuresis is ineffective. Isopropyl alcohol and acetone are water soluble and are removed well by hemodialysis, which should be considered in patients with levels exceeding 400 mg/dL or in patients who do not respond well to conservative therapy.

References

Alexander CB, McBay AJ, Hudson RP. Isopropanol and isopropanol deaths—ten years' experience. *J Forensic Sci.* 1982;27:541-548

Lacouture PG, Heldreth DD, Shannon M, Lovejoy FH Jr. The generation of acetonemia/acetonuria following ingestion of a subtoxic dose of isopropyl alcohol. *Am J Emerg Med.* 1989;7:38-40

Lacouture PG, Wason S, Abrams A, Lovejoy FH Jr. Acute isopropyl alcohol intoxication: diagnosis and management. *Am J Med.* 1983;75:680-686

Natowicz M, Donahue J, Gorman L, Kane M, McKissick J, Shaw L. Pharmacokinetic analysis of a case of isopropanol intoxication. *Clin Chem.* 1985;31:326-328

Rosansky SJ. Isopropyl alcohol poisoning treated with hemodialysis: kinetics of isopropyl alcohol and acetone removal. *J Toxicol Clin Toxicol.* 1982;19:265-271

Lead

Available Forms and Sources: Lead is a ubiquitous environmental toxin and is a common cause of chronic poisoning in children (Table 17). Significant symptomatic single exposures to lead are uncommon. Because of the toxicity of lead, particularly to the central nervous system, public health efforts have been organized to identify affected children, to develop plans for management, and to reduce the amount of lead in the environment.

Table 17. Common Sources of Lead*

High Dose	Intermediate Dose	Low Dose
Interior/exterior paint	Dust (household)	Food
	Interior renovation	Ambient air
	Contaminated soil	Drinking water
	Industrial sources	

*Adapted from 1987 AAP policy statement on childhood lead poisoning.

The most common source of lead in children is from lead-based paint in the form of chips or dust. Lead concentrations in paint were not uniformly reduced to safe levels until 1978, and most housing built before 1950 in the United States is assumed to contain some lead-based paint. Lead is still a constituent of automobile, marine, and military paint. Flaking or shed paint chips are accessible to curious, ambulatory toddlers and are described as sweet. Children with excessive oral behaviors (pica) may also chew on window or crib frames, ingesting lead-based paint from formerly intact surfaces (including those that are covered by lead-free paint).

Lead-based paint can become pulverized into dust, which creates a secondary source of lead. Lead-based dust is typically found in high concentration around window wells and door frames. It may also be produced during any indoor or outdoor household renovation (eg, scraping or demolition). Ingested lead dust is more efficiently absorbed than paint chips; dust may also be absorbed upon inhalation. If a parent encounters lead at work (eg, contractors or smelter workers), it can be brought into the home on work clothes and contaminate a previously lead-free environment.

Soil may contain high concentrations of lead, both as a result of paint that falls from the exterior of homes as well as by contamination from atmospheric lead released from automobile and industry emissions. While a safe lead concentration in soil is considered <300 ppm, urban areas may have concentrations in excess of 5000 ppm. Soil may become a significant source of lead in children with pica.

Another potential source of lead in children is from the ingestion of lead-contaminated water. Until recently public water sources were required to maintain a maximum contaminant level of lead of ≤50 µg/L (50 parts per billion [ppb]). The maximum contaminant level has been replaced by an action level of 15 ppb, which was designed to further reduce the lead concentration in public waters. However, because of the widespread use of lead pipes until the 1950s and the sanctioned use of lead-based solder until 1986, many residential plumbing circuits contain leechable lead. Residential tap water and water fountains in schools may contain lead concentrations in excess of 100 ppb. The highest lead concentrations occur in the first-drawn water of the day and in hot water. The lead concentration of water may be further increased if lead-containing water is boiled in a vessel that contains lead.

With the exception of water, there are few significant dietary sources of lead. Cans that contain a lead solder seam may bring lead in direct contact with food. Lead may also contaminate food or juices if they are stored in containers that are lead based (eg, imported pottery with ceramic glazes or Middle Eastern cooking urns). Certain vegetables, particularly the dark, leafy variety, contain lead if grown in soil with a high lead content. Ingestion of large, lead-containing foreign bodies (fishing or curtain weights) that are retained in the gastrointestinal tract can also add to significant lead absorption.

Lead is readily transmitted across the placenta, with lead levels in the blood of the fetus being 75% to 100% of maternal levels. In pregnant women who have significant levels of lead (generally from occupational sources or an improper home renovation), congenital intoxication may occur.

Certain cosmetics and folk remedies contain lead, including Greta and Azarcon, popular remedies for treating gastrointestinal illnesses in Mexico and Latin America, and Surma, an Asian cosmetic. If these remedies are administered to children, lead intoxication may result.

Substance abuse in children and adolescents has also been associated with lead intoxication. The synthesis of methamphetamine includes a reaction requiring the addition of lead acetate, which may not be completely removed in the final stages of production. Gasoline sniffing may cause organic lead intoxication if leaded gasoline is used.

Acute lead intoxication is unusual but almost always occurs by inhalation, leading to severe clinical toxicity, including death. The creation of lead fumes by burning objects that contain lead (eg, batteries) or by using a heat gun to remove paint during home renovation can lead to sudden, dramatic rises in levels of lead in the blood.

Mechanism of Toxicity and Signs and Symptoms: Lead

has a number of toxicologic properties affecting the renal, skeletal, hematopoietic, and nervous systems.

Since lead is actively accumulated in the kidneys, it produces nephrotoxicity and eventual renal insufficiency. Lead-associated hypertension may occur in adults as a result of childhood plumbism. Lead also affects skeletal development, primarily through renal injury, which impairs the conversion of 25-hydroxyvitamin D to 1,25-dihydroxyvitamin D. Chronic lead intoxication causes decreased bone growth, which may be associated with the appearance of lines of growth arrest ("lead lines") on radiography. Lead is not a cause of short stature. Because bone is the major repository for in situ lead storage, illnesses associated with prolonged immobilization and associated bone resorption can result in elevations in levels of lead in the blood in children with prior lead intoxication.

Lead affects several enzymes in the heme synthetic pathway. Inhibition of the enzyme ferrochelatase leads to elevations in levels of the heme precursor erythrocyte protoporphyrin. Only severe lead intoxication impairs heme synthesis enough to produce frank anemia (although anemia is commonly found in lead-poisoned children as a result of concurrent iron deficiency). Severe lead intoxication is also occasionally associated with the appearance of basophilic stippling.

Lead affects the peripheral and central nervous systems. The primary effect on the peripheral nervous system is a peripheral neuropathy (which may be subclinical). Lead has its most pronounced effects in the central nervous system. Because proliferation and maturation of central nervous system neurons are maximal in early childhood, exposure to lead during this age may cause significant neurodevelopmental injury. Nerve cells exposed to lead are hypoplastic, with decreased dendritic arborization and diminished production of neurotransmitters. With low-level lead intoxication these effects may be associated with subtle disturbances in cognitive function (eg, mild learning disabilities). Moderate to severe lead exposure can cause severe global delays in neurodevelopment (mental retardation). Severe lead intoxication, in addition to causing neurodevelopmental injury, may also cause an encephalopathy that includes headaches, irritability, somnolence, coma, seizures, cerebral edema, and death.

Other reported clinical manifestations of lead intoxication include abdominal pain ("lead colic"), constipation, and eosinophilia.

Toxic Dose: Lead balance studies in infants have found that daily exposures of >5 μg/kg can result in a positive lead balance with resultant increases in the blood lead level.

A classification of toxic blood lead concentrations in children has been established by the Centers for Disease Control and Prevention and is designed to tailor patient treatment to the degree of lead exposure (Table 18).

Diagnostic Testing: Lead screening is the cornerstone of diagnostic testing. Lead is not detected in a routine drug screen. Children at high risk for lead exposure (those living in housing built before the 1950s, those with pica, those with siblings or close friends with plumbism, and those who live with adults exposed to lead at work) should receive lead screening regularly. Children at low risk should also be screened but not as frequently. Although universal lead screening was formerly accomplished by capillary sampling of blood for measurement of zinc protoporphyrin (ZPP), this has proven to be an insensitive measure of low-level lead exposure. Therefore, only the direct measurement of lead can be utilized for the identification of children with significant levels of lead in their blood. Although capillary lead measurements are acceptable for screening purposes, false elevations can occur if the technique is not scrupulous. If the capillary blood lead level is elevated, confirmation should be performed with blood obtained by venipuncture.

Table 18. Classification of Blood Lead Levels in Children*

Blood Lead, μg/dL	Classification	Recommended Intervention
≤ 9	I	None
10-14	IIa	Community intervention No pharmacologic therapy Repeat blood lead determinations in 3 mo
15-19	IIb	Individualized case management Environmental counseling Nutritional assessment/supplementation No pharmacologic therapy Repeat blood lead determinations in 3 mo
20-44	III	Medical referral Environmental inspection/lead abatement Nutritional assessment/supplementation Consider pharmacologic intervention
45-69	IV	Environmental inspection/lead abatement Pharmacologic intervention Consider hospitalization
≥ 70	V	Hospitalization Pharmacologic intervention Environmental inspection/lead abatement

*Based on confirmatory blood lead level.
Adapted from the Centers for Disease Control and Prevention, October 1991.

General Treatment: Treatment of elevated levels of lead in the blood begins with identification of the primary source and efforts at reducing further exposure. According to the Centers for Disease Control and Prevention guidelines, if large numbers of children have levels of 10 to 14 μg/dL, management is based on community efforts to reduce lead concentration. With levels of 15 to 19 μg/dL, an individualized care plan is initiated by the pediatrician or health care provider, which includes discussion with parents about common sources of environmental lead and instruction on methods to reduce dust (eg, frequent cleaning with high-phosphate detergent). Also, there should be a nutritional assessment with attention to the child's intake of iron and calcium. If deficiency in any of these nutrients is found or suspected, empiric supplementation should be provided. No pharmacologic intervention is instituted; levels of lead, however, should be obtained again in 3 months to determine the effect of intervention.

Children with levels of lead between 20 and 44 µg/dL may require medical referral to a program with expertise in treating children with lead intoxication. Environmental inspection, particularly for lead-based paint or dust, should be performed. With lead levels in this range, it is likely that a source of lead will be found. If lead is found in accessible areas on interior or exterior surfaces, a plan for lead abatement should be outlined. Pharmacologic therapy may be necessary for levels of lead in this range.

Children with levels of lead of ≥45 µg/dL require pharmacologic intervention. These children may require hospitalization, both for the administration of medication as well as for environmental protection because levels ≥45 µg/dL generally indicate a significantly at-risk environment for the child. An environmental inspection should be conducted, and high-dose sources of lead should be removed or alternate housing found as soon as possible. If the child is hospitalized, lead hazards should be identified and removed prior to returning to the environment.

Decontamination: (Refer to the treatment section p 6 for the appropriate use of these techniques.) Because of the slow and incomplete absorption of lead, gastric emptying is not necessary with lead exposure. Lead does not bind to activated charcoal. Cathartics or whole bowel irrigation may be used to remove paint chips from the intestinal tract prior to chelation therapy.

Antidote: Several chelating agents are available for the treatment of lead intoxication (see Table 2, p 16, for specific dosing).

BAL in oil (dimercaprol) is a chelator generally reserved for blood lead levels >70 µg/dL and acts primarily by chelating erythrocyte-bound lead, enhancing its elimination through urine and bile. Because the vehicle for BAL is peanut oil, it is only administered intramuscularly. The administration of BAL in oil is associated with a high rate of adverse effects including cardiovascular disturbances, a metallic taste in the mouth, and pain at the injection site. It should not be administered simultaneously with oral iron therapy.

Edetate calcium disodium ($CaNa_2EDTA$) is a chelator that promotes the urinary elimination of lead. EDTA is used both diagnostically (the EDTA lead mobilization test) and therapeutically and is most effective in children with blood lead levels >45 µg/dL. At lower levels of lead in the blood, EDTA may not promote an effective lead diuresis. Therefore, in children with levels of lead 25 to 45 µg/dL, the lead mobilization test identifies those who will have a satisfactory response to EDTA therapy. In performing the lead mobilization test the child is given a single injection (intramuscular or intravenous) of EDTA, followed by a 6- to 8-hour urine collection. Total urinary lead excretion is expressed as a fraction of the dose of EDTA administered:

$$\frac{\text{Total urinary lead (µg)}}{\text{Total EDTA dose (mg)}}$$

A ratio of >0.5 to 0.6 is considered positive for lead poisoning and suggests that additional doses of EDTA should be administered. A negative mobilization test suggests that EDTA will be relatively ineffective. The lead mobilization test is painful if the injections are given intramuscularly. Urine collection may be problematic if the child is not toilet trained, and test results may be uninterpretable if urine is spilled. The EDTA mobilization test has diminishing importance with the recognition of the limited range of efficacy of EDTA.

When the EDTA lead mobilization test is positive or blood lead levels are >45 µg/dL, EDTA is given in 3- to 5-day or more courses. It may be given twice daily, preferably by intravenous injection. However, because of its rapid elimination half-life, EDTA is ideally administered by continuous infusion. A "rebound," or increase in levels of blood lead occurs after EDTA therapy, reflecting redistribution of lead from soft tissue into blood.

Succimer (dimercaptosuccinic acid, DMSA) is an oral congener of dimercaprol and is highly effective in reducing levels of lead in the blood by more than 75% with 5 days of therapy. Currently succimer is approved for use in children with levels of lead ≥45 µg/dL (although preliminary data suggest that it has an identical profile of safety and efficacy with levels of lead <45 µg/dL). Succimer is given in a fixed, 19-day course that includes a 5-day therapeutic period. Completion of a 19-day course of succimer is often associated with a substantial rebound in levels of lead in the blood. The rebound may necessitate multiple courses of therapy to effect sustained reductions in levels of lead in the blood. Adverse reactions to succimer include reversible abnormalities in liver function and the white blood cell count.

d-Penicillamine is an oral agent that is also used as a chelator of lead and appears to remove lead from blood, soft tissue, and bone. d-Penicillamine is not FDA approved for use in the treatment of lead intoxication in children, although there is substantial experience with its use. Succimer is probably the preferred agent. d-Penicillamine may cause several mild adverse reactions including nausea, mild, reversible depression of the white blood cell and platelet counts, allergic-type dermal eruptions, and hematuria. The overall rate of significant adverse reactions is 10%. Like dimercaprol, d-penicillamine should not be administered concomitantly with oral iron therapy.

Although much of the management of childhood plumbism can be provided on an outpatient basis, general criteria for hospital admission include (1) blood lead levels >50 to 60 µg/dL; (2) sudden increases in levels of lead in the blood, signifying a lead-contaminated environment; or (3) an abnormal abdominal radiograph. Hospital admission permits aggressive gastrointestinal decontamination, chelation, and provides a lead-free environment. Children with levels of lead >70 µg/dL should receive combination chelation therapy with dimercaprol and EDTA. Levels <70 µg/dL may be treated with either intravenous EDTA or oral succimer. Children should be kept in the hospital until lead hazards have been eliminated or reduced or alternate housing is found.

For children with levels of lead in their blood that do not warrant hospitalization, chelation therapy can be provided under an outpatient protocol. Generally, pharmacologic therapy is reserved for those with lead levels that consistently remain above 20 µg/dL. Current Centers for Disease Control and Prevention guidelines recommend the lead mobilization test for children with levels of 25 to 44 µg/dL. If the lead mobilization test is negative, alternate therapies should be considered.

Patient Monitoring: All treatment regimens require frequent monitoring of levels of lead in the blood, renal function, and adverse reactions. Tests of renal function should include a urinalysis and determinations for serum urea nitrogen and serum creatinine. Because many of the children are also iron deficient, it is important to perform a serum iron, total iron-binding capacity, ferritin, and a complete blood count with mean corpuscular volume.

Radiographs may be of some utility in the initial evaluation of a child with known or suspected lead intoxication. In cases in which a history of paint chip ingestion is given (or suspected), an abdominal radiograph may identify the presence of radiodense material. If the material is present, a cathartic agent should be administered to prevent its systemic absorption. Abdominal radiographs generally are not clinically useful in cases in which the presumed mode of exposure is dust inhalation. Low-level exposures to lead (blood lead levels <30 µg/dL) are rarely associated with abnormal radiographs. A single anteroposterior radiograph of the knee may demonstrate the presence of growth arrest lines in the proximal fibula. Growth arrest lines suggest but are not diagnostic of chronic, moderate to severe plumbism. Artifactual dense lines in the distal femur or proximal tibia may result from their larger dimensions.

Neuropsychological testing, although ideal, is difficult to perform during initial assessment and may give unreliable information. It should be considered at the end of treatment.

Specific Treatment: Treatment is supportive. There is no specific treatment.

Enhanced Elimination: Dialytic techniques are of no proven value.

References

General

Agency for Toxic Substances and Disease Registry. *The Nature and Extent of Lead Poisoning in Children in the United States: A Report to Congress.* Atlanta, GA: Public Health Service; 1988. US Dept of Health and Human Services publication DHHS 99-2966

American Academy of Pediatrics, Committee on Environmental Health. Lead poisoning: from screening to primary prevention. *Pediatrics.* 1993;92:176-183

Centers for Disease Control. *Preventing Lead Poisoning in Young Children: A Statement by the Centers for Disease Control.* Atlanta, GA; 1991

Hu H. A 50-year follow-up of childhood plumbism—hypertension, renal function, and hemoglobin levels among survivors. *AJDC.* 1991;145:681-687

Markowitz ME, Weinberger HL. Immobilization-related lead toxicity in previously lead-poisoned children. *Pediatrics.* 1990;86:455-457

Shannon M, Graef JW. Hazard of lead in infant formula. *N Engl J Med.* 1992;326:137

Shannon M, Graef JW. Lead intoxication in infancy. *Pediatrics.* 1992; 89:87-90

Shannon M, Lindy H, Anast C, Graef JW. Recurrent lead poisoning in a child with immobilization osteoporosis. *Vet Hum Toxicol.* 1988;30:586-588

Sharp DS, Becker CE, Smith AH. Chronic low-level lead exposure—its role in the pathogenesis of hypertension. *Med Toxicol.* 1987;2:210-232

Neurodevelopmental Effects

Bellinger D, Leviton A, Slomon J. Antecedents and correlates of improved cognitive performance in children exposed in utero to low levels of lead. *Environ Health Perspect.* 1990;89:5-11

Bellinger D, Sloman J, Leviton A, Rabinowitz M, Needleman HL, Waternaux C. Low-level lead exposure and children's cognitive function in the preschool years. *Pediatrics.* 1991;87:219-227

Dietrich KN, Krafft KM, Bornschein RL, et al. Low-level fetal lead exposure effect on neurobehavioral development in early infancy. *Pediatrics.* 1987;80:721-730

Faust D, Brown J. Moderately elevated blood lead levels: effects on neuropsychologic functioning in children. *Pediatrics.* 1987;80:623-629

McMichael AJ, Baghurst PA, Wigg NR, Vimpani GV, Robertson EF, Roberts RJ. Port Pirie cohort study: environmental exposure to lead and children's abilities at the age of four years. *N Engl J Med.* 1988;319:468-475

Needleman HL, Schell A, Bellinger D, Leviton A, Allred EN. The long-term effects of exposure to low doses of lead in children—an 11-year follow-up report. *N Engl J Med.* 1990;322:83-88

Needleman HL, Gatsonis CA. Low-level lead exposure and the IQ of children: a meta-analysis of modern studies. *JAMA.* 1990;263:673-678

Shukla R, Dietrich KN, Bornschein RL, Berger O, Hammond PB. Lead exposure and growth in the early preschool child: a follow-up report from the Cincinnati lead study. *Pediatrics.* 1991;88:886-892

Environmental/Nutritional Interventions

Amitai Y, Brown MJ, Graef JW, Cosgrove E. Residential deleading: effects on the blood lead levels of lead-poisoned children. *Pediatrics.* 1991;88: 893-897

Amitai Y, Graef JW, Brown MJ, Gerstle RS, Kahn N, Cochrane PE. Hazards of "deleading" homes of children with lead poisoning. *AJDC.* 1987;141:758-760

EDTA

Kassner J, Shannon M, Graef JW. Role of forced diuresis on urinary lead excretion after the ethylenediaminetetraacetic acid mobilization test. *J Pediatr.* 1990;117:914-916

Markowitz ME, Rosen JF. Assessment of lead stores in children: validation of an 8-hour $CaNa_2EDTA$ provocative test. *J Pediatr.* 1984;104:337-341

Markowitz ME, Rosen JF. Need for the lead mobilization test in children with lead poisoning. *J Pediatr.* 1991;119:305-310

Shannon M, Grace A, Graef JW. Use of urinary lead concentration in interpretation of the EDTA mobilization test. *Vet Hum Toxicol.* 1989;31:140-142

Weinberger HL, Post EM, Schneider T, Helu B, Friedman J. An analysis of 248 initial mobilization tests performed on an ambulatory basis. *AJDC.* 1987;141:1266-1270

Penicillamine

Shannon M, Grace A, Graef JW. Use of penicillamine in children with small lead burdens. *N Engl J Med.* 1989;321:979-980

Shannon M, Graef JW, Lovejoy FH Jr. Efficacy and toxicity of d-penicillamine in low-level lead poisoning. *J Pediatr.* 1988;112:799-804

Succimer

Graziano JH, Lolacono NJ, Meyer P. Dose-response study of oral 2,3-dimercaptosuccinic acid in children with elevated blood lead concentrations. *J Pediatr.* 1988;113:751-757

Graziano JH, Lolancono NJ, Moulton T, Mitchell ME, Salokovich U, Zarate C. Controlled study of meso-2,3 dimercaptosuccinic acid for the management of childhood lead intoxication. *J Pediatr.* 1992;110:133-139

Mercury

Available Forms and Sources: Mercury may be found in three general forms—elemental mercury in thermometers, batteries, and pressure gauges; inorganic mercury as many different salts; and organic mercury in Merthiolate and contaminated food and water.

Mechanism of Toxicity: All three forms of mercury are toxic. Organic mercury compounds and elemental mercury are converted into inorganic mercury (mercuric ion) in the body. Organic mercury is lipid soluble and distributes widely into tissues, most notably the brain and nerve tissue. Both organic and inorganic forms of mercury have a high affinity for sulfhydryl compounds and produce cellular toxicity by binding to sulfhydryl groups of enzymes. Signs of inorganic mercury toxicity probably result from both inhibition of catechol-O-methyl transferase, the enzyme responsible for catecholamine metabolism and direct neurotoxicity. Mercury is a renal tubular toxin.

Toxic Dose: Mercury is a cumulative toxin. The duration of exposure as well as the dose determines the severity of symptoms and progression of illness. Ingestion of as little as 0.2 g of mercuric chloride has resulted in death in a child. Because small amounts of elemental mercury, such as that contained in a household thermometer, are poorly absorbed, toxicity after ingestion is unlikely. Acute systemic toxic reactions from organic mercury compounds such as Merthiolate are unlikely unless massive amounts are ingested.

Signs and Symptoms: Mercury toxicity may occur after short- and long-term exposure. Symptoms in either case depend on the form of mercury involved in the exposure. Elemental mercury is poorly absorbed from the gastrointestinal tract. Symptomatic exposures usually occur after inhalation of vapors from heated or spilled mercury. Initial acute symptoms include headache, fever, respiratory symptoms, and a metallic taste in the mouth. Symptoms may progress to encephalopathy. Nausea, diarrhea, and abdominal cramps may also occur. Long-term exposure can cause acrodynia (pink disease) and nephrotic syndrome. Acrodynia is a symptom complex that includes rashes, irritability, tachycardia, hypertension, anorexia, poor muscle tone, and swelling and redness of the hands and feet. Acrodynia can occur after exposure to elemental or inorganic mercury.

Inorganic mercury salts are corrosive to the gastrointestinal tract. Symptoms include oral burning, nausea, vomiting (often heme positive), and abdominal pain. Shock and renal failure may occur. Chronic poisoning produces multi-organ system symptoms. Dermatoses, gingivitis, stomatitis, and gastrointestinal symptoms are common. Central nervous system symptoms include insomnia, irritability, timidity, anxiety, and memory loss. Intention tremors, gait disturbances, and clonus may be seen. Renal failure may lead to death.

The symptoms of poisoning with organic mercurials depend on the specific compound. The organic mercury in Merthiolate produces symptoms similar to those seen with inorganic mercurials. Methylmercury produces a neuroencephalopathy manifested with dysarthria, ataxia, and visual field constriction (Minamata disease).

Diagnostic Testing: Mercury is not detected on a routine drug screen. Whole blood mercury levels are the best measure of short-term exposure to mercury. Levels exceeding 2 µg/dL generally reflect significant exposure. After chronic exposure, mercury is excreted into the urine, but the amount excreted does not correlate with the severity of symptoms. Urinary concentrations above 30 µg of mercury per liter suggest excessive exposure. Individuals without identifiable or excessive exposure excrete less than 20 µg of mercury per liter of urine. Blood mercury values decline rapidly after exposure and are usually not as helpful to evaluate chronic exposure unless there is renal impairment.

General Treatment: Therapy is generally supportive. Exposure to the source of mercury should be discontinued, which may be sufficient treatment for mild or asymptomatic cases. Supportive care may include antihypertensive therapy and clinical management of renal insufficiency or failure.

Decontamination: (Refer to the treatment section p 6 for the appropriate use of these techniques.) Emesis may be helpful following large short-term exposures but is of no value following chronic exposures. Activated charcoal treatment is probably of no value.

Antidote: Several chelating agents have been used to treat mercury poisoning, although conclusive data on their effectiveness in humans are lacking (see Table 2, p 16, for specific dosing). Therapy using BAL in oil (dimercaprol) has been advocated following severe inorganic mercury poisoning, although a newer derivative DMSA (2,3-dimercaptosuccinic acid; succimer) may be more effective. Succimer is not approved by the FDA for treatment of mercury poisoning. Another derivative, DMPS, is currently investigational. d-Penicillamine also has been used in less severe exposures, although conclusive data of its effectiveness are also lacking. Organic or elemental mercury poisoning should not be treated using BAL in oil.

Specific Treatment: Treatment is supportive. There is no specific treatment.

Patient Monitoring: Renal function should be monitored. For patients experiencing gastrointestinal symptoms, levels of electrolytes should be monitored.

Enhanced Elimination: Enhanced elimination techniques are of no proven value.

References

Boyer Hassen LV, Dart RC, Arthur AW, Hurlbut KM. Subacute toxicity in a family exposed to elemental mercury vapor, and the use of dimercaptosuccinic acid in their treatment. *Vet Hum Toxicol.* 1992;34:353

Fagan DG, Pritchard JS, Clarkson TW, Greenwood MR. Organ mercury levels in infants with omphaloceles treated with organic mercurial antiseptic. *Arch Dis Child.* 1977;52:962-964

Kark RAP, Poskanzer DC, Bullock JD, Boylen G. Mercury poisoning and its treatment with N-acetyl-D,L-penicillamine. *N Engl J Med.* 1971; 285:10-16

Lien DC, Todoruk DN, Rajani HR, Cook DA, Herbert FA. Accidental inhalation of mercury vapour: respiratory and toxicologic consequences. *Can Med Assoc J.* 1983;129:591-595

Powell PP. Minamata disease: a story of mercury's malevolence. *South Med J.* 1991;84:1352-1358

Rohyans J, Walson PD, Wood GA, MacDonald WA. Mercury toxicity following Merthiolate ear irrigations. *J Pediatr.* 1984;104:311-313

Methanol (Methyl Alcohol)

Available Forms and Sources: Methanol, sometimes called wood alcohol, can be found in many household products including paint removers and strippers (3% to 28%), glass cleaners (1% to 38%), model engine fuel (43% to 77%), pipe sweetener (75%), brake fluid (<4%), carburetor fluid (99%), gasoline antifreeze (100%), windshield deicer (4% to 89%), windshield washer solution (17% to 99%), and gasohol (10%).

Mechanism of Toxicity: Methanol is metabolized by the hepatic alcohol dehydrogenase pathway to formaldehyde and formic acid. Formic acid, the principal toxic metabolite, inhibits mitochondrial respiration, which results in tissue hypoxia and metabolic (lactic) acidosis. Formic acid is converted to carbon dioxide by folate-dependent enzymes. Visual impairment and optic nerve damage are well-known toxic sequelae and are probably produced by formic acid. Hypoglycemia can result from impaired gluconeogenesis.

Toxic Dose: Ingestion is the most common route of exposure, but significant absorption can occur dermally and via inhalation, especially in poorly ventilated spaces. Toxicity has been reported with ingestion of 0.4 mL/kg of 100% (absolute) methanol. A dose of 15 mL of 40% methanol (6 mL of 100%) has been fatal. Patients initially seen with levels of serum bicarbonate <20 mEq/L have an almost 20% mortality; those with levels of <10 mEq/L have up to 50% mortality.

Signs and Symptoms: Initially there may be no symptoms, or only inebriation and drowsiness. Signs of toxicity may be delayed up to 72 hours after exposure because methanol metabolism is relatively slow. In young infants, metabolism may be even slower, and symptoms may be delayed beyond 72 hours. Methanol produces central nervous system depression. After a delay of 12 to 24 hours, severe acidosis and visual disturbances may develop. Other signs include nausea, vomiting, dysphoria, abdominal pain, headache, weakness, and dizziness. Lethargy and confusion occur with moderate intoxication. In severe intoxication, coma and seizures are caused by cerebral edema. Adults have reported cloudy or blurred vision, constricted visual fields, decreased acuity, or scotomata (a feeling of "being in a snow storm"). Children may not be able to relate or describe visual disturbances. Permanent visual impairment may occur after severe poisonings, despite appropriate therapy. Other findings include unreactive, dilated pupils, retinal edema, and optic disc hyperemia. Hyperpnea is associated with severe metabolic acidosis. Death results from myocardial depression, bradycardia, hypotension, shock, and respiratory arrest. Laboratory assessment reveals low levels of serum bicarbonate, a low pH, and an increased anion gap and osmolal gap (see p 28 for toxicity calculations).

Diagnostic Testing: Methanol is detected in some routine drug screens. If methanol levels are not readily available, the freezing point depression osmolality can be used to estimate the osmolal gap (p 28). The osmolal gap can then be used to estimate the blood methanol level as follows:

$$\text{ESTIMATED BLOOD METHANOL LEVEL} = \text{OSMOLAL GAP} \times 3.2$$
(in mg/dL, or mg%)

If another alcohol or ethylene glycol was also ingested, blood methanol levels cannot be reliably estimated using this method. Blood methanol levels do not correlate with visual disturbances or permanent visual impairment. Formic acid levels correlate with the severity of intoxication but are usually not available. Obtain serum electrolyte levels and calculate the anion gap.

General Treatment: Because significant symptoms are possible, the need for life support measures including respiratory support should be anticipated. Ethanol infusion and dialysis may be needed.

Decontamination: (Refer to the treatment section p 6 for the appropriate use of these techniques.) Emesis should not be used because methanol is rapidly absorbed and central nervous system depression may occur. Gastric lavage may be useful if instituted within 30 to 60 minutes after ingestion. Activated charcoal does not bind methanol and should not be used. For dermal exposures, the skin should be washed thoroughly after removal of any contaminated clothing. For inhalation exposures, move the person to fresh air.

Antidote: Ethanol is the preferred substrate for alcohol dehydrogenase and inhibits methanol metabolism, increasing the elimination half-life of methanol to 30 to 35 hours. Ethanol therapy is indicated for symptomatic patients if the amount ingested is estimated to be more than 0.4 mL/kg (absolute, or 100% methanol), if the blood methanol level is 20 mg/dL or higher, or if metabolic acidosis is present (see p 28 for toxicity calculations) **(see Table 2, p 16, for specific dosing).** Ethanol loading is also recommended in symptomatic patients who are awaiting hemodialysis or the results of methanol determination. After ethanol loading, repeated dosing (oral or nasogastric) or continuous intravenous infusion of ethanol should be started. Oral ethanol may cause nausea or emesis. Intravenous infusion is the most reliable route of administration, but phlebitis may occur, and many hospitals may not stock intravenous ethanol. Blood ethanol levels should be monitored at least every 2 hours and the dose adjusted to maintain the blood ethanol level at 100 to 150 mg/dL. Folate administration to enhance formic acid metabolism is experimental, but folic acid, 50 mg administered intravenously every 4 hours for several days, has been used safely in adults. 4-Methylpyrazole is an experimental drug that inhibits alcohol dehydrogenase and prevents methanol metabolism but is currently not commercially available.

Specific Treatment: Metabolic acidosis should be treated with intravenous sodium bicarbonate at doses of 2 to 3 mEq/kg. Hypoglycemia is treated with 2 to 3 mL/kg of 25% dextrose intravenously, followed by a 5 mL/kg/h infusion of 10% dextrose. Intravenous fluids should be administered to replace urinary losses and correct electrolyte imbalance and hypotension. Seizures can be treated with benzodiazepines **(see Table 3, p 22, for specific dosing).**

Patient Monitoring: Monitor electrolytes, glucose, serum urea nitrogen, and serum transaminase levels. Arterial blood gases are helpful to determine the need for ventilatory support in severe intoxications.

Enhanced Elimination: Hemodialysis is indicated for refractory metabolic acidosis, visual disturbances, or blood methanol levels >50 mg/dL. Ethanol therapy should be continued during hemodialysis and requires an increase in the dose to maintain a blood ethanol level of 100 to 150 mg/dL.

References

Brent J, Lucas M, Kulig K, Rumack BH. Methanol poisoning in a 6-week-old infant. *J Pediatr.* 1991;118:644-646

Burkhart KK, Kulig KW. The other alcohols. *Emerg Med Clin North Am.* 1990;8:913-928

Litovitz T. The alcohols: ethanol, methanol, isopropanol, ethylene glycol. *Pediatr Clin North Am.* 1986;33:311-323

Naphthalene

Available Forms and Sources: Naphthalene is a colorless crystalline hydrocarbon. Although its use has declined, it is still found in some home deodorizers and mothballs or moth cakes. It is also used as a chemical intermediate and in veterinary products.

Mechanism of Toxicity: The primary toxicity of naphthalene relates to the metabolite α-naphthol, which can cause methemoglobinemia and hemolysis of the red blood cells. These effects are most prominent in newborns and those with glucose-6-phosphate dehydrogenase (G6PD) deficiency.

Toxic Dose: The toxic dose in susceptible individuals is probably 10 to 15 g, although it is not well defined.

Signs and Symptoms: Naphthalene ingestion may lead to gastrointestinal irritation. Dysuria may occur, and urine may be brown secondary to the excretion of naphthalene metabolites.

Acute hemolytic anemia occurs in newborns and G6PD-deficient patients. The onset of hemolytic anemia may be delayed 1 to 3 days. Methemoglobinemia has also been reported. Central nervous system symptoms may occur but are thought to be secondary to severe anemia with tissue hypoxia. Jaundice may also be seen due to the hemolytic process.

Diagnostic Testing: Naphthalene is not detected in routine drug screens. Naphthalene-containing mothballs can be distinguished from the more common varieties containing paradichlorobenzene based on the difference of their specific gravity. Mothballs containing naphthalene float in a saturated solution of table salt. Mothballs containing paradichlorobenzene sink in this salt solution.

General Treatment: Significant acute symptoms are not anticipated.

Decontamination: (Refer to the treatment section p 6 for the appropriate use of these techniques.) Emesis can be used if instituted soon after the exposure. Gastric lavage with activated charcoal or activated charcoal treatment alone may also be used.

Antidote: No specific antidotes are available.

Specific Treatment: If acute hemolytic anemia develops, treat the patient with alkaline diuresis to prevent renal damage and blood transfusions as necessary.

Patient Monitoring: In patients who have ingested large amounts of naphthalene, G6PD status should be assessed. Alternatively, these patients can be followed up by obtaining one or more hemoglobin measurements on days 1 and 3 following ingestion. A methemoglobin level should be obtained only if methemoglobinemia is suspected.

Enhanced Elimination: Enhanced elimination techniques are of no proven value.

References

Fukuda T, Koyama K, Yamashita M, Koichi N, Takeda M. Differentiation of naphthalene and paradichlorobenzene mothballs based on their difference in specific gravity. *Vet Hum Toxicol.* 1991;33:313-314

Valaes T, Doxiadis SA, Fessas P. Acute hemolysis due to naphthalene inhalation. *J Pediatrics.* 1963;63:904-915

Zuelzer WW, Apt L. Acute hemolytic anemia due to naphthalene poisoning: clinical and experimental study. *JAMA.* 1949;141:185

Paradichlorobenzene

Available Forms and Sources: Paradichlorobenzene (PDB) is the most commonly used chemical in diaper pail deodorizers and toilet bowl deodorizer cakes. This substance is also found in moth repellent products such as mothballs, flakes, cakes, and crystals.

Mechanism of Toxicity: Paradichlorobenzene is oxidized in the liver primarily to sulfate and glucuronide conjugates. A small amount of PDB is converted to epoxide intermediates, which can cause hepatic necrosis.

Toxic Dose: Dichlorobenzene compounds have a low degree of acute and chronic toxicity. Paradichlorobenzene is absorbed through the gastrointestinal tract as well as by inhalation. Enteral absorption is enhanced in the presence of milk or food high in fat. A toxic dose in children has not been established. A lethal oral dose is estimated to be approximately 500 to 5000 mg/kg. A mothball containing PDB weighs about 5 g.

Signs and Symptoms: Although patients are frequently asymptomatic, nausea, vomiting, and diarrhea may occur. One case report of methemoglobinemia, hemolytic anemia, and jaundice in a 3-year-old has been described. Irritation of the eyes and nose can occur. Inhalation can irritate the upper respiratory tract.

Diagnostic Testing: Paradichlorobenzene is not detected by most drug screens. No accurate diagnostic test for PDB exists. The urinary metabolite 2,5-dichlorophenol has been used as an index of exposure in occupational cases, but this measurement is not widely available. Mothballs containing PDB can be distinguished from the more toxic and seldom used mothballs containing naphthalene on the basis of specific gravity. Mothballs containing PDB sink in a saturated solution of table salt, whereas mothballs containing naphthalene float.

General Treatment: Symptomatic care is usually adequate because significant symptoms are unlikely to occur.

Decontamination: (Refer to the treatment section p 6 for the appropriate use of these techniques.) Emesis can be used if instituted early after exposure. Gastric lavage and/or activated charcoal may also be used.

Antidote: No specific antidotes are available.

Specific Treatment: Avoid milk or fatty foods for at least 2 hours after ingestion. If acute hemolytic anemia develops, treat the patient with alkaline diuresis to prevent renal damage and blood transfusions as necessary.

Patient Monitoring: A complete blood count should be obtained only if hemolytic anemia is suspected. A methemoglobin level should be obtained only if methemoglobinemia is suspected.

Enhanced Elimination: Enhanced elimination techniques are of no proven value.

References

Blumer JL, Reed MD. Mothball toxicity. *Pediatr Clin North Am.* 1986; 33:369-374

Fukuda T, Koyama K, Yamashita M, Koichi N, Takeda M. Differentiation of naphthalene and paradichlorobenzene mothballs based on their difference in specific gravity. *Vet Hum Toxicol.* 1991;33:313-314

Hallowell M. Acute haemolytic anaemia following the ingestion of paradichlorobenzene. *Arch Dis Child.* 1959;34:74-75

Loeser E, Litchfield MH. Review of recent toxicology studies on p-dichlorobenzene. *Food Chem Toxicol.* 1983;21:825-832

Winkler JV, Kulig K, Rumack BH. Mothball differentiation: naphthalene from paradichlorobenzene. *Ann Emerg Med.* 1985;14:30-32

Paraquat and Diquat

Available Forms and Sources: Paraquat and diquat are non-selective bipyridyl herbicides sold under various trade names including Ortho Paraquat and Gramoxone.

Mechanism of Toxicity: Toxicity is thought to involve the production of free radical oxygen (superoxide radicals) and, secondarily, interference with nicotinamide-adenine dinucleotide phosphate (NADP) and NADPH (the reduced form of NADP) metabolism. Cellular injury occurs primarily in the lung following paraquat ingestion and primarily in the gastrointestinal tract and kidneys following diquat ingestion, resulting in organ dysfunction. Paraquat-induced pulmonary fibrosis results from alveolar injury.

Toxic Dose: Death has occurred following ingestion of 2 g (10 mL of 20% concentrate) of paraquat in an adult and is common following ingestion exceeding 40 mg/kg. The toxic dose in children is not defined.

Signs and Symptoms: Initial symptoms following paraquat ingestion include nausea, vomiting, diarrhea, and oral mucous membrane irritation, which occur during the first 24 hours after ingestion and resolve within a few days. Following paraquat (but not diquat) ingestion, pulmonary function deteriorates beginning several days after exposure, resulting in irreversible pulmonary fibrosis in fatal cases. When large amounts of paraquat (>10 g) have been ingested, severe emesis with fluid and electrolyte imbalances have occurred. Cardiac and renal dysfunction and cerebral edema may develop, with death occurring within 48 hours after ingestion.

Paralytic ileus may occur following diquat ingestion. Renal failure develops over the first few days after ingestion, with recovery possible within 2 weeks. Intracranial hemorrhage and parkinsonian-like syndrome have also been observed. Dermal irritation is common. Sufficient amounts of paraquat may be absorbed following prolonged dermal contact to produce systemic toxicity including death.

Oral and nasal irritation with epistaxis may occur after inhalation. There are no reports of systemic toxic reactions resulting from inhalation without ingestion or prolonged dermal contact.

Diagnostic Testing: These agents are not routinely identified in a drug screen. Serum or urinary paraquat levels, if available, may serve to confirm exposure and to provide prognostic information.

General Treatment: Because significant acute symptoms are possible, aggressive supportive care should be available. The administration of supplemental oxygen is *not recommended* unless it is necessary to sustain life.

Decontamination: (**Refer to the treatment section p 6 for the appropriate use of these techniques.**) Emesis may be desirable if induced rapidly (within 30 to 60 minutes) after ingestion and is not otherwise contraindicated. Activated charcoal or adsorbent clay (Fuller's Earth) may be administered.

Antidote: No specific antidotes are available.

Specific Treatment: Anti-inflammatory agents (corticosteroids or immunosuppressants) and free radical scavengers have had no significant effect in the treatment regimens tried to date.

Patient Monitoring: Monitor renal function, electrolyte status, and measures of oxygenation and ventilation (such as arterial blood gases or pulse oximetry).

Enhanced Elimination: Hemoperfusion should be performed if the patient is initially seen within the first 2 to 6 hours after ingestion of paraquat. Hemoperfusion against charcoal or resin cartridges appears to be the most effective means of enhancing elimination. Hemodialysis is relatively ineffective.

References

Pond SM. Manifestations and management of paraquat poisoning. *Med J Aust.* 1990;152:256-259

Wohlfahrt DJ. Fatal paraquat poisonings after skin absorption. *Med J Aust.* 1982;1:512-513

Vanholder R, Colardyn F, DeReuck J, Praet M, Lameire N, Ringoir S. Diquat intoxication: report of 2 cases and review of the literature. *Am J Med.* 1981;70:1267

Polychlorinated Biphenyls (PCBs) and Dioxin

Available Forms and Sources: Polychlorinated biphenyls (PCBs) are mixtures of chlorinated biphenyl congeners. Manufacturing of PCBs ceased in the 1970s and their use in new products has been banned. Polychlorinated biphenyls were used in electrical transformers, heat exchangers, and capacitors. 2,3,7,8-Tetrachlorodibenzodioxin (TCDD, or dioxin) is one of many tricyclic polychlorinated compounds that are contaminants of some agricultural or industrial chemical processes, or are produced in the combustion of PCBs, chlorinated plastics (eg, polyvinyl chloride), and other chlorinated compounds. Dioxin is also used as a generic term to refer to dibenzodioxins and dibenzofurans, which are related polychlorinated compounds. Polychlorinated biphenyls and dioxin persist in the environment and bioaccumulate in the food chain, resulting in widespread "background" human exposure. Human exposure occurs primarily by consumption of fish, dairy products, and meat. Polychlorinated biphenyls and dioxin are lipid soluble and are excreted into breast milk.

Mechanism of Toxicity: Polychlorinated biphenyls and dioxin induce cytochrome P450 hepatic enzymes. Dioxin is especially potent and may act as a hormone by binding to a cytoplasmic receptor protein (the "Ah" receptor), which then moves into the cell nucleus and alters cell function. At high doses dioxin produces a wasting syndrome in animals. Immunosuppression also occurs, which is especially prominent in immature animals or with prenatal exposure. Dioxin is an animal teratogen, producing renal anomalies, cleft palate, and behavioral abnormalities. In animals, PCBs and dioxin may promote hepatocellular tumors and other carcinomas.

Toxic Dose: Polychlorinated biphenyls and dioxins have not been proven to be clinically toxic to humans under conditions of usual environmental or dietary exposure. Species and sex sensitivity to dioxin varies greatly, with humans being less susceptible than nonhuman primates and guinea pigs, two species that show reproductive toxic reactions at low levels (10^{-9} to 10^{-12} g/d).

Signs and Symptoms: Clinical symptoms from dioxin have been described after chronic occupational exposure or releases of high levels into the environment. The only finding consistently associated with such exposure to dioxin is chloracne, a cystic acneiform rash on the arms, trunk, and legs as well as the face, neck, and back. Elevations in levels of serum transaminases or triglycerides and induction of hepatic enzymes have been inconsistently noted. Similar PCB exposure has not produced consistent findings. To date carcinogenic effects in humans have not been convincingly demonstrated, and federal regulatory agencies classify PCBs and dioxin as "potential" human carcinogens.

A common problem in studies of PCBs or dioxin health effects in humans is that when exposure occurs, mixtures of PCBs or mixtures of dioxins are often present, as well as other toxic contaminants (such as dibenzofurans). Highly publicized epidemics resulted from consumption of PCB-contaminated rice oil in Japan and Taiwan, but dioxins and highly toxic dibenzofurans were also contaminants in the oil, so the relationship of PCBs to the illness is unclear. Symptoms reported from this exposure included chloracne, brown pigmentation of the nails and skin, conjunctivitis, fever, and weakness. At birth, infants with in utero exposure were growth retarded and had brown pigmentation of the mucous membranes and skin, natal teeth, and scalp edema. Skin color faded to normal after 2 to 5 months, but infants were developmentally delayed. Similar dermal changes have been noted in other industrial releases of PCBs or in fires involving PCBs that resulted in mixed PCB, dioxin, and dibenzofuran exposure.

Prenatal exposure to PCBs from maternal consumption of heavily contaminated fish has inconsistently been associated with slightly decreased birth weight and head circumference. Mild motor impairments were noted in infants with higher cord blood levels of PCBs, but these effects were transient. Developmental delay or impairment has not been associated with the low levels of PCBs that result from background exposure.

Diagnostic Testing: These agents are not detected in routine drug screens. Polychlorinated biphenyls or dioxin levels in blood or fat are neither widely available nor clinically useful.

General Treatment: No medical treatment is available or indicated for environmental or dietary exposures to PCBs or dioxin. Unnecessary exposure can be avoided by compliance with fish or wildlife advisories and avoiding consumption of fish or animals known to be contaminated. The benefits of breast-feeding outweigh theoretical risks to the infant unless a mother is known to have excessive PCB or dioxin body stores.

Decontamination: (**Refer to the treatment section p 6 for the appropriate use of these techniques.**) Although ingestion of significant amounts is uncommon, it can be treated with emesis, gastric lavage, or activated charcoal. Dermal exposures should be washed with soap and water followed by a lipid solubilizing agent if needed.

Antidote: No specific antidotes are available.

Specific Treatment: Treatment is supportive. There is no specific treatment.

Patient Monitoring: No specific monitoring is necessary.

Enhanced Elimination: Enhanced elimination techniques are of no proven value.

References

Ames BN. Natural carcinogens and dioxin. *Sci Total Environ.* 1991; 104:159-166

Fein GG, Jacobson JL, Jacobson SW, Schwartz PM, Dowler JK. Prenatal exposure to polychlorinated biphenyls: effects on birth size and gestational age. *J Pediatr.* 1984;105:315-320

Gladen BC, Rogan WJ. Effects of perinatal polychlorinated biphenyls and dichlorodiphenyl dichloroethane on later development. *J Pediatr.* 1991; 119:58-63

Kimbrough RD. Consumption of fish: benefits and perceived risk. *J Toxicol Environ Health.* 1991;33:81-91

Kimbrough RD. How toxic is 2,3,7,8-tetrachlorodibenzodioxin to humans? *J Toxicol Environ Health.* 1991;30:261-271

Lilienfeld DE, Gallo MA. 2,4-D, 2,4,5-T, and 2,3,7,8-TCDD: an overview. *Epidemiol Rev.* 1989;11:28-58

Lione A. Polychlorinated biphenyls and reproduction. *Reproductive Toxicol.* 1988;2:83-89

Tilson HA, Jacobson JL, Rogan WJ. Polychlorinated biphenyls and the developing nervous system: cross-species comparisons. *Neurotoxicol Teratol.* 1990;12:239-248

Radon

Available Forms and Sources: Radon is a naturally occurring radioactive gas present in outside and indoor air. It results from the decay of trace amounts of uranium in soil. Radon radioactive decay releases alpha particles. Radon gas is colorless and odorless.

Mechanism of Toxicity: Release of alpha particles at local lung tissue levels results in an increased risk for lung cancer.

Toxic Dose: The risk of lung cancer increases with the dose deposited in the lungs, which is directly related to the concentration in air. The risk of dying from lung cancer due to a lifetime of radon exposure at a level of 4 pCi/L of air is approximately equivalent to smoking half a pack of cigarettes per day. Radioactive decay products of radon may cause 25% of the lung cancers in nonsmokers over age 60 years. The Environmental Protection Agency recommends that indoor air home concentrations of radon not exceed 4 pCi/L. Average outdoor levels are about 0.3 pCi/L of air. Highest indoor air levels are usually found in basements. The decay half-life is about 4 days.

Signs and Symptoms: The signs and symptoms are the same as those of lung cancer. The latency period for the development of disease after exposure exceeds 20 years.

Diagnostic Testing: State and local health departments may offer testing kits to measure air levels of radon. Various filter systems and adsorbents (eg, activated charcoal) are used to trap radon from air passed through the collection device, which is then returned to a laboratory for analysis. If elevated levels are found, abatement should be considered.

General Treatment: Prevention of exposure is the only effective measure. Effective reduction of exposure sometimes may be as simple as increasing the ventilation in a basement or other area.

Decontamination: Decontamination is not applicable for this type of exposure.

Antidote: No specific antidotes are available.

Specific Treatment: Treatment is supportive. There is no specific treatment.

Patient Monitoring: No monitoring is necessary.

Enhanced Elimination: Enhanced elimination techniques are of no proven value.

References

Ames BN, Magaw R, Gold LS. Ranking possible carcinogenic hazards. *Science*. 1987;236:271-280

Council on Scientific Affairs. Radon in homes. *JAMA*. 1987;258:668-672

Samet JM, Nero AV. Indoor radon and lung cancer. *N Engl J Med*. 1989; 320:591-594

Rodenticides - Anticoagulants

Available Forms and Sources: Most rodenticides in common use contain anticoagulants. Many contain the short-acting anticoagulant warfarin in a concentration of 0.05% mixed in corn meal or seed. "Superwarfarins" are long-acting warfarin derivatives developed to counteract warfarin resistance among rodents. These derivatives include brodifacoum, chlorphacinone, difenacoum, and diphacinone.

Other types of rodenticides, including arsenic, red squill, strychnine, thallium, and zinc phosphate, are less commonly used and are not included in this discussion.

Mechanism of Toxicity: Toxic reactions are induced by inhibition of the hepatic enzyme vitamin K_1-2,3-reductase, thereby blocking synthesis of vitamin-K-dependent clotting factors (II, VII, IX, and X).

Toxic Dose: Warfin toxicity requires the ingestion of either a massive dose or multiple smaller doses over several days to produce anticoagulation. The single toxic dose is highly variable. The usual therapeutic dose is 0.2 mg/kg/d; single doses five times that amount, however, are unlikely to produce clinically significant bleeding.

Superwarfarin toxicity has been reported following a single ingestion of 0.12 mg/kg of brodifacoum.

Signs and Symptoms: Clinical signs and symptoms result from hemorrhaging and vary depending on the site of bleeding. If bleeding is severe, shock from blood loss may develop. Intracranial bleeding, gastrointestinal hemorrhage, retroperitoneal bleeding, hemarthroses, and epistaxis have all been reported. Clinical bleeding is usually observed more than 48 to 72 hours after ingestion because prothrombin time (PT) inhibition does not begin until 24 to 36 hours after ingestion.

Diagnostic Testing: These agents are not detected in a routine drug screen. Serum anticoagulant levels are not of value in making an acute diagnosis.

General Treatment: Significant symptoms are not anticipated.

Decontamination: (Refer to the treatment section p 6 for the appropriate use of these techniques.) Emesis can be used if initiated early. Gastric lavage with activated charcoal, or activated charcoal treatment alone may also be used. Most exposures do not require treatment.

Antidote: Administration of clotting factors usually corrects the factor deficiency. After severe poisonings, however, large amounts may be necessary to correct an apparent consumptive coagulopathy. Vitamin K administration (as phytonadione, vitamin K_1) in large doses competes with the ingested vitamin K inhibitor **(see Table 2, p 16, for specific dosing)**. After superwarfarin poisoning, very large doses of oral phytonadione (40 mg/kg or more) may be required on a daily basis for weeks to months.

Specific Treatment: Supportive care only is needed.

Patient Monitoring: Measure the patient's PT and hemoglobin level or hematocrit value. In most cases, the optimal time for PT measurement is 36 to 60 hours after ingestion. If symptoms are present or a large amount of rodenticide has been ingested, measurement of the patient's PT at presentation, 24 hours, and 48 hours after ingestion is appropriate. Partial thromboplastin time (PTT) is generally not prolonged except in severe poisonings.

Enhanced Elimination: Enhanced elimination techniques are of no proven value.

References

Katona B, Wason S. Superwarfarin poisoning. *J Emerg Med.* 1989;7: 627-631

Smolinske SC, Scherger DL, Kearns PS, Wruk KM, Kulig KK, Rumack BH. Superwarfarin poisoning in children: a prospective study. *Pediatrics.* 1989;84:490-494

BIOLOGICAL TOXINS

Hymenoptera Envenomations

Available Forms and Sources: The hymenoptera are a group of arthropods including bees, wasps, and ants.

Mechanism of Toxicity: In general, the mechanism of toxicity associated with hymenoptera envenomation is a hypersensitivity reaction. The venoms associated with these arthropods contain a number of peptides that may cause histamine release (via mast cell degranulating peptide), necrosis of muscle, and intravascular hemolysis, Some species of ants in addition to stinging can bite leaving saliva containing formic acid and other irritants that may produce inflammation.

Toxic Dose: A single exposure may produce an anaphylactic reaction. Multiple stings or bites may also cause direct toxicity by cumulative effects of the venom.

Signs and Symptoms: Signs and symptoms can be divided into two general categories. The acute hypersensitivity reactions include typical signs of angioedema, upper airway obstruction, hypotension, respiratory failure, hives, flushing, and pruritus. There may also be a delayed effect that resembles a serum sickness reaction following exposure to these venoms. The second pattern of envenomation is generally associated with large, multiple doses of venom and includes edema, respiratory failure, hypotension, and renal failure. Widespread damage to muscle can occur, causing rhabdomyolysis and renal failure. Intravascular hemolysis has also been reported.

Diagnostic Testing: No diagnostic testing is available for the effects of venom. In patients who have had an IgE-specific response, however, experimental assays of specific IgE may suggest the presence of hypersensitivity reaction ir some historical cases.

General Treatment: Cardiorespiratory compromise should be anticipated in patients with a known allergy or multiple stings.

Decontamination: Stingers that are retained in the skin should be scraped off rather than removed with forceps or by other methods. Scraping off the stinger prevents further venom exposure by not squeezing the venom sack on the end of a stinger. Wash the affected area with soap and an antiseptic.

Antidote: No specific antidotes are available.

Specific Treatment: Hypersensitivity reactions can be treated systematically using epinephrine subcutaneously for milder envenomations or intravenously for more life-threatening situations. Aminophylline and β_2-agonist aerosols may be useful for the management of acute bronchospasm. Antihistamines such as diphenhydramine and corticosteroids should be administered for any systemic manifestations **(see Table 3, p 22, for specific dosing)**. The long-term prevention of hypersensitivity reactions by the use of immunotherapy or management by the patient by carrying epinephrine injections is somewhat controversial, but referral to individuals trained in treatment of allergic manifestations may be appropriate.

　　The treatment for multiple stings is largely supportive, because no specific antivenin is available. Because of the possibility of non-IgE mediated histamine release complicating the acute massive exposure to venom, antihistamine therapy should be considered even without other manifestations of a hypersensitivity reaction.

Patient Monitoring: In cases where large doses of venom have been injected, renal function should be assessed and urine examined for myoglobinuria. Arterial blood gases should be monitored if respiratory compromise occurs.

Enhanced Elimination: Enhanced elimination techniques are of no proven value.

References

Banner W. Bites and stings in the pediatric patient. *Curr Probl Pediatr.* 1988;18:1-69

Chipps BE, Valentine MD, Kagey-Sobotka A, Schuberth KC, Lichtenstein LM. Diagnosis and treatment of anaphylactic reactions to hymenoptera stings in children. *J Pediatr.* 1980;97:177-184

Marine Envenomation

Available Forms and Sources: The topic of marine envenomations is too varied to be comprehensively addressed in a short text. Large numbers of exotic species may produce severe life-threatening reactions, particularly in the Indo-Pacific waters. The more commonly encountered envenomations by physicians in North America are from marine aquariums or shallow waters near the Atlantic coast and include lionfish, stingray, jellyfish, and coral. A discussion of the toxicology and treatment for each of these envenomations follows. Food poisoning due to ingested fish may occur as ciguatera (from grouper, red snapper, and others), tetrodotoxin (from puffer fish), or scombroid poisoning (from tuna, bonito, mahi-mahi, and others). It will not be discussed in this text.

Mechanism of Toxicity: Toxic effects are due to complex venoms with highly variable effects.

Toxic Dose: The toxic doses for these venoms are not known.

Signs and Symptoms and General Treatment: Controlled data are lacking on the most effective approach to the management of marine envenomations, and most of the information presented is anecdotal. Because venoms from the marine environment may produce anaphylactic reactions or may contain histamine-releasing materials, supportive care of severe exposures may involve treatment for anaphylaxis.

Lionfish. The lionfish is a member of the scorpaenidae family, in which some other members are known to possess lethal venom. The spine of the lionfish, however, contains venom that produces toxicity that is not generally life threatening. Systemic effects including hypotension, muscle weakness, and respiratory compromise have been reported. The major symptom is severe pain.

Most sources recommend immersion of the envenomated area in hot water (45°C) in order to inactivate the venom until symptoms resolve. Other therapies have been suggested, including the use of papain (an ingredient in meat tenderizer), and a variety of other cleansing types of remedies. The wound should be treated as if it is contaminated with respect to surgical management.

Stingrays. Stingrays tend to feed and live in shallow, sandy bottoms in water that is often used by people for recreational activities and are therefore a fairly common source of envenomation. Although stingrays are not aggressive, if they are stepped on they respond by inflicting a wound with their tail stinger that is traumatic as well as venomous. The wound should be considered contaminated with respect to surgical management and carefully followed for secondary infection. Suturing may be needed in rare cases for structural or cosmetic reasons. Cleanse the wound carefully and inspect the wound for foreign bodies including the venom apparatus. In general, a painful wound is the only manifestation, but systemic effects have been noted and may be severe, including abdominal pain with nausea and vomiting, muscle cramps and fasciculations, hypotension, tachycardia, and headache.

Treatment is controversial and includes vigorous irrigation of the wound with the most readily available solution followed by immersion in hot water at 45°C for 30 to 90 minutes to inactivate the venom.

Jellyfish. "Jellyfish" is a general term for a variety of nematocyst-containing invertebrates that range from the uniformly lethal box jellyfish to smaller species that are only mild contact irritants. The most famous jellyfish is the *Physalia,* also known as the Portuguese man-of-war.

Nematocysts are small structures with coiled stinging mechanisms that are triggered by contact to strike and release venom. Because of the large number of nematocysts that are present in the tentacles of the jellyfish, large amounts of venom may be released. The venom of the man-of-war contains histaminergic components, potentially causing an IgE-mediated hypersensitivity reaction. Initial management includes the treatment of anaphylaxis.

Other intervention focuses on removal and neutralization of the remaining nematocysts using either a weak acetic acid solution (vinegar) or an aluminum sulfate surfactant solution. Rinsing the wound with alcohol to denature the remaining nematocyst has been recommended, but may cause nematocysts to discharge. Other treatment includes the use of antihistamines, bronchodilators, and support for cardiovascular manifestations that may rarely occur.

Corals. Some corals, particularly fire coral, may produce a similar nematocyst form of envenomation. The most common symptom is intense local pain with a burning sensation. It is unlikely that systemic manifestations will develop, and treatment is focused on the local reaction. Some sources recommend the use of a vinegar solution or isopropyl alcohol followed by vigorous cleansing of the area and treatment with a steroid cream to decrease inflammation.

Sea Urchins. All species of sea urchins have sharp spines that are capable of producing mechanical trauma and irritation upon contact. Few species produce a true envenomation. Symptoms are usually intense local pain followed by a slow resolving inflammatory process. Systemic symptoms including nausea, weakness, muscle spasm, and light-headedness occur infrequently.

Wounds should be thoroughly cleansed, with careful attention to removing residual spines. Pain responds to immersion in hot water (45°C). Systemic symptoms are treated with supportive care.

Antidote: Antivenin treatment as a specific modality is only available for certain sea snakes, box jellyfish, and stonefish. All of these species are generally found in the Indo-Pacific region and are unlikely to be found in the United States. Commercial antivenin for these envenomations is not available in the United States.

References

Auerbach PS. Hazardous marine animals. *Emerg Med Clin North Am.* 1984;2:531-544

Bengston K, Nichols MM, Schnadig V, Ellis MD. Sudden death in a child following jellyfish envenomation by *Chiropsalmus quadrumanus:* case report and autopsy findings. *JAMA.* 1991;266:1404-1406

Burnett JW, Calton GJ. Jellyfish envenomation syndromes updated. *Ann Emerg Med.* 1987;16:1000-1005

Ikeda T. Supraventricular bigeminy following a stingray envenomation: a case report. *Hawaii Med J.* 1989;48:162

Mushrooms

Available Forms and Sources: Identification of mushrooms cannot be easily done over the telephone, and a local mycologist should be consulted. The need for urgent identification depends on many variables, including the prevalence of dangerous species in the geographical area involved, the habitat in which the mushrooms were found, and the quantity ingested; thus, no specific nationwide protocol for handling poisonous mushroom ingestion exists. Consultation with a regional poison center is suggested.

Mechanism of Toxicity: Mushrooms produce seven known syndromes and the mechanism of toxicity depends on the toxin or toxins present. Table 19 lists characteristic signs, symptoms, onset of symptoms, mechanism of toxicity, and specific treatment for each toxin.

Toxic Dose: The toxic dose is highly variable and depends on the toxin.

Signs and Symptoms: Gastroenteritis may be the only complaint of an otherwise benign ingestion or part of many other syndromes. Therefore, emesis is not recommended because it may mask this important sign. If gastroenteritis occurs identification of the mushroom should be pursued. Other syndromes of poisoning include potentially lethal hepatotoxicity, (cyclopeptides; monomethylhydrazine), an "Antabuse-like" reaction (coprine), cholinergic crisis (muscarine), delirium or hallucinations (muscimol, ibotenic acid, psilocybin), anticholinergic syndrome (ibotenic acid, muscimol), and renal failure (orelline).

Diagnostic Testing: Mushroom identification should be attempted in all symptomatic cases. Specimens, either those partially ingested or obtained from the same geographic area, should be kept in a paper bag in the refrigerator. Gastric contents and

Table 19. Mushroom Poisoning Syndromes

Group	Toxin/Mechanism	Representative Species	Common Name	Onset	Signs/Symptoms	Treatment
I	Amatoxins (amanitine)/ interferes with RNA polymerase II-mediated transcription	*Amanita phalloides* *Galerina autumnalis*	Death cap ...	6-24 h 36-48 h	Abdominal pain, vomiting, profuse bloody or mucoid diarrhea Hepatitis	Forced diuresis, electrolyte replacement, penicillin G 300 000-1 000 000 U/kg/d IV Silibinin (investigational)
Ia	Orelline, Cortinarin A and B/tubulo-interstitial nephritis due to alkaline phosphatase inhibition	*Cortinarius orellanus*	...	36 h to 20 d	Gastroenteritis, headache, chills, night sweats, tinnitus, somnolence, thirst, oliguria, chronic renal failure	Hemodialysis and/or hemoperfusion
II	Muscimol, ibotenic acid, muscazone/ mimics GABA at receptor site, peripheral anticholinergic activity	*Amanita muscaria* *Amanita pantherina*	Fly agaric Panther	30-90 min 4-6 h	Dry, hot, flushed skin, drowsiness, confusion, euphoria, dizziness, ataxia, muscle spasms, delirium, visual illusions Deep sleep/coma lasting 4-8 h, seizures	Supportive care, symptomatic treatment

Table 19. Mushroom Poisoning Syndromes *(continued)*

Group	Toxin/Mechanism	Representative Species	Common Name	Onset	Signs/Symptoms	Treatment
III	Monomethyl hydrazine/ inhibits pyridoxine-dependent step in GABA synthesis	*Gyromitra esculenta*	False morel	2-8 h (inhalation) 6-12 h (ingestion) 2-6 d	Bloating, vomiting, watery diarrhea, headache, leg cramps, abdominal pain Jaundice, methemoglobinemia, vertigo, seizures, coma, delirium, mydriasis	Pyridoxine 25 mg/kg IV for neurological symptoms, hydration, electrolyte replacement
IV	Muscarine, histamine/ attaches strongly to acetylcholine receptor site causing prolonged stimulation	*Inocybe geophylla* *Omphalotus olearius* (also known as *Clitocybe illudens*)	White inocybe Jack O'Lantern	30-120 min	Cholinergic crisis - perspiration, sali- vation, lacrimation, miosis, bradycardia, abdominal pain, diarrhea, hypotension, bronchospasm	Atropine, 0.05 mg/kg test dose; repeat if needed to end point (cessation of secretions)
V	Coprine/inhibits aldehyde dehydrogenase	*Coprinus atramentarius*	Inky cap	20 min- 2 h	Nontoxic if ingested alone. Disulfiram-like reaction if ingested before or within 72 h of alcohol ingestion (nausea, vomiting, palpitations, pares- thesias, facial flushing, metallic taste, malaise)	Supportive care, symptomatic treatment

	Mechanism/Toxin	Species	Common name	Onset	Symptoms	Treatment
VI	Psilocybin, psilocin/ stimulates autonomic nervous system and serotonin receptors	*Conocybe cyanopus*	...	30-60 min	Visual, sensory, space and time distortion, nausea, vomiting, mydriasis, facial flushing, tachycardia, hypertension ataxia, febrile seizures, hyperreflexia, panic reactions	Reassurance, diazepam orally for panic reactions, antipyretics
		Gymnopilus spectabilis	Big laughing mushroom			
		Panaeolus cyanescens	Blue meanies			
		Psilocybe cubensis	Magic mushroom			
VII	Sesquiterpenes, norcaperatic acid, lectins, hemagglutinins/ mechanism diverse, gastro-intestinal irritants	*Boletus sensibilis*	...	30-120 min	Vomiting, abdominal cramps, diarrhea, chills, paresthesias	Hydration and electrolyte replacement
		Chlorophyllum molybdites	Green parasol			
		Gomphus flocculus	...			
		Hebeloma mesophallium	...			
		Lactarius piperatus	...			
		Entoloma lividum	...			
		Russula emetica	...			
		Scleroderma citrinum	The sickener			
		Tricholoma pardinum	Pig skin poison			

stools should be saved and refrigerated for spore identification in potentially severe cases.

General Treatment: Supportive care is most important.

Decontamination: (**Refer to the treatment section p 6 for the appropriate use of these techniques.**) If ingestion of a potentially deadly mushroom is suspected, many sources recommend inducing emesis even though it masks early gastrointestinal symptoms. Treatment with activated charcoal may be as effective and is preferred.

Antidote: Few antidotes exist; the toxin should preferably be identified before the administration of an antidote (see Table 19).

Specific Treatment: Specific drug intervention is rarely required, and care is symptomatic.

Patient Monitoring: Liver and renal function should be monitored following ingestions of mushrooms that may affect these organs.

Enhanced Elimination: Hemodialysis may be required for supportive care if hepatic or renal failure develops; it is not used to remove the toxin.

References

McCormick DJ, Avbel AJ, Gibbons RB. Nonlethal mushroom poisoning. *Ann Intern Med.* 1979;90:332-335

Rumack BH, Salzman E, eds. *Mushroom Poisoning: Diagnosis and Treatment.* Boca Raton, FL: CRC Press; 1978

Plants

Available Forms and Sources: Plants constitute the fourth most common exposure category reported by poison centers. Over 80% of the plant exposures occur in children younger than 6 years.

More than 700 known poisonous plants exist in the northern hemisphere, but only the most common ones are listed in Table 20. Nontoxic plants and berries are listed in Tables 5 and 6, pp 32-33.

Mechanism of Toxicity: The specific mechanisms and toxic constituents of plants are listed in Table 20.

Toxic Dose: The toxic dose of a plant is highly variable and may depend on the part of the plant ingested and the cultivation and habitat of the plant. Many berries and seeds must be thoroughly chewed to release toxic material.

Signs and Symptoms: Even if plant parts do not contain toxic constituents, they are a foreign body aspiration and digestive hazard for small children. Dermatitis is the most common symptom reported following plant exposures. The most common cause of contact dermatitis is poison ivy. Mouth irritation, nausea, and vomiting also frequently occur. Specific symptoms are listed in Table 20.

Diagnostic Testing: Most plant constituents cannot be measured in body fluids. They are not detected as such in routine toxicology screens.

General Treatment: Remove any plant material from the mouth and airway.

Decontamination: (Refer to the treatment section p 6 for the appropriate use of these techniques.) The ingestion of plants can irritate the mouth and gastrointestinal tract, and administering cool fluids may provide symptomatic relief. Emesis or activated charcoal therapy should be considered if a potentially toxic amount has been ingested. Gastric lavage may have limited value in removing large pieces of plant material.

Table 20. Poisonous Plants

Plants	Scientific Name	Toxic Part or Ingredient	Symptoms and Special Treatment
Houseplants and Cultivated Flowers			
Philodendron Caladium Dumb cane Elephant ear Peace lily Pothos	*Philodendron* sp *Caladium* sp *Dieffenbachia* sp *Colocasia* sp *Spathiphyllum* sp *Epipremnum aureum*	Oxalates	Irritation of the buccal mucosa, edema of the pharynx, gastroenteritis; large ingestions may result in hypocalcemia. **Treatment:** rinse the mouth with milk; use calcium salts for systemic hypocalcemia (see Table 3, p 22)
Narcissus Amaryllis Daffodil	All are subfamily *Amaryllidaceae*	The alkaloid lycorine	Vomiting and diarrhea
Lily-of-the-Valley Foxglove Oleander	*Convallaria majalis* *Digitalis purpurea* *Nerium oleander*	Cardiac glycosides	Irritation of the mucous membranes, cardiovascular toxicity. **Treatment:** measure serum potassium level and treat if high (digoxin-specific Fab fragments [Digibind], bicarbonate, glucose, insulin [see Table 2, p 16]); further drugs and therapies appropriate to electrocardiogram findings
Monkshood Larkspur	*Aconitum* sp *Delphinium* sp	Alkaloid aconitine	Restlessness, salivation, irregular heartbeat. **Treatment:** gastric decontamination
Autumn crocus Glory lily	*Colchicum autumnal* *Gloriosa* sp	Colchicine	Gastrointestinal, respiratory, renal, and central nervous system toxicity

Poinsettia Snow-on-the-mountain	*Euphorbia* sp	Unknown acrid principle in milky sap	Irritation of mucous membranes and gastrointestinal tract. Poinsettia usually not toxic
Anemone	*Anemone* sp	Protoanemonin aglycone	Irritation to mucous membrane, gastroenteritis
Iris	*Iris* sp	Resins like podophyllotoxin	Gastroenteritis
Jerusalem cherry	*Solanum pseudocapsicum*	Solanine alkaloids	Gastroenteritis, central nervous system depression
Aloe	*Aloe* sp	Latex contains anthraquinones	Oral irritation, nausea, vomiting, diarrhea
Christmas pepper	*Capsicum annum*	Capsicum	Strong irritant; stinging and burning of mucous membranes
Chrysanthemum	*Chrysanthemum* sp	Sesquiterpene lactones, pyrethrins	Skin reactions

Plants Found as Wild Flowers and Weeds

Deadly nightshade Black nightshade Climbing nightshade (also called woody or deadly) Jimson weed Henbane	*Atropa belladonna* *Solanum nigrum* *Solanum dulcamara* *Datura* sp *Hyoscyamus niger*	Atropine, solanine, and related glycoalkaloids Anticholinergic alkaloids	Dry mouth; mydriasis and loss of accommodation; hot, flushed skin; hyperthermia; convulsions. **Treatment:** emesis; physostigmine for severe anticholinergic symptoms (seizures, hallucinations, hypertension, dysrhythmias) (see antidote chart, Table 2, p 16)

Table 20. Poisonous Plants *(continued)*

Plants	Scientific Name	Toxic Part or Ingredient	Symptoms and Special Treatment
Horse nettle	*Solanum carolinense*	Solanine alkaloid	Gastroenteritis, central nervous system depression
Green hellebore False hellebore	*Veratrum viride Veratrum californicum*	Veratrum alkaloids	Gastrointestinal irritation; respiratory and cardiovascular depression. **Treatment:** atropine (see antidote chart, Table 2, p 16)
Death camus	*Zygadenus venenous*	Veratrum alkaloids	Nausea, vomiting, hypotension, bradycardia, syncope, paresthesias, weakness, electrocardiogram changes. **Treatment:** atropine (see antidote chart, Table 2, p 16)
Pokeweed	*Phytolacca sp*	Resins like podophyllotoxins	Vomiting, sweating, colic, diarrhea, central nervous system depression
May apple	*Podophyllum* sp	Podophylloresin	May produce peripheral neuropathy, vomiting, colic, diarrhea, drowsiness, impaired vision
Poison ivy Poison oak Poison sumac Poison wood	*Toxicodendron sp*	Urushiol	Dermatitis manifested by red, itchy skin and clear blisters that exude serum; if ingested, causes severe mucosal irritation. **Treatment:** 1% hydrocortisone lotion or calamine lotion, systemic steroids if mucosa is severely irritated
Spurges	*Euphorbia sp*	Unknown acrid principle	Severe irritation to mucosa

Common name	Scientific name	Toxin	Symptoms / Treatment
Jack-in-the-pulpit Wild calla Skunk cabbage	*Arisaema triphyllum Calla palustris Symplocarpus foetidus*	Calcium oxalate crystals	Irritation and burning of the mouth. **Treatment:** rinse mouth with milk or magnesium hydroxide
Water hemlock	*Cicuta maculata*	Cicutoxin	Grand mal seizures. **Treatment:** symptomatic to prevent and control seizures, salivation, vomiting, and diarrhea
Poison hemlock	*Conium maculatum*	Alkaloid coniine	Salivation, nausea, vomiting, diarrhea, sensory disturbances, seizures, coma; death may occur from respiratory paralysis. **Treatment:** symptomatic
White snakeroot	*Eupatorium rugosum*	Tremetol, may be in the milk of a poisoned cow	Weakness, debilitation, vomiting, tremors, and death
Precatory bean (rosary pea)	*Abrus precatorius*	Phytotoxin abrin	Burning sensation of the mouth and throat, delayed gastroenteritis, depression of vasomotor center, vascular collapse
Buttercup Morning glory	*Ranunculus sp Ipomoea violaceae*	Protoanemonin Seeds contain lysergic acid monoethylamide	Gastrointestinal irritation Central nervous system and psychic stimulation

Plants Grown in Gardens and as Cultivated Crops

Potato Tomato	*Solanum tuberosum Lycopersicum esculentum*	Foliage (tomatoes, potatoes), and sprouts contain solanine alkaloids	Gastrointestinal irritation, headache, and central nervous system depression, dermatitis

Table 20. Poisonous Plants *(continued)*

Plants	Scientific Name	Toxic Part or Ingredient	Symptoms and Special Treatment
Rhubarb	*Rheum rhaponticum*	Leaves contain oxalate crystals and soluble oxalates	Irritation of oral and gastric mucosa; ingestion results in hypocalcemia with seizures. **Treatment:** rinse mouth with milk; use intravenous calcium salts for hypocalcemia (see Table 3, p 22)
Tobacco	*Nicotiana sp*	Nicotine	Salivation, gastroenteritis; large amounts produce convulsions
Castor bean	*Ricinus communis*	Toxalbumin ricin - must be chewed to release toxic material	Burning sensation of the mouth and throat, delayed gastroenteritis, depression of vasomotor center, hepatic injury, hemolysis, convulsions, and death
Plants Found as Trees and Woody Shrubs			
Cherry trees Apple trees Peach trees Apricot trees Choke cherry trees	*Prunus sp Malus sylvestria Prunus persica Prunus armeniaca Prunus virginiana*	Leaves and pits or seeds contain glycosides hydrolyzed to hydrocyanic acid - must be chewed to release cyanogenic material	Dyspnea, paralysis, convulsions, coma, and death. **Treatment:** emesis, sodium nitrite intravenously; see antidote chart, Table 2, p 16, for cyanide therapy.
Mountain laurel Rhododendrons	*Kalmia latifolia Rhododendron sp*	Grayanotoxin	Local and gastrointestinal irritation, respiratory and cardiovascular depression. **Treatment:** atropine (see antidote chart, Table 2, p 16)

Yew	*Taxus* sp	Alkaloid taxine	Vomiting, colic, hypotension, respiratory depression
English holly	*Ilex aquifolium*	Ilexanthin and ilex acid	Vomiting and diarrhea
Mistletoe	*Phoradendron flavescens*	Berries contain lectins, phoratoxin, viscotoxin, polysaccharides	Gastroenteritis and cardiovascular collapse
Black locust	*Robinia pseudoacacia*	Toxalbumin	Anorexia, weakness, gastroenteritis, dilated pupils, weak and irregular pulse
Daphne	*Daphne* sp	Glycoside in which the aglycone is dihydrohycoumarin	Burning and irritation to the skin and gastrointestinal tract, bloody diarrhea, stupor, weakness, and convulsions

Antidote: A few specific antidotes for plant poisoning are listed in the Table.

Specific Treatment: Specific treatments are listed in the table and are based on the anticipated symptoms.

Patient Monitoring: Monitor vital signs and laboratory values as dictated by the plant and potential symptoms.

Enhanced Elimination: Enhanced elimination techniques are of no proven value.

References

Lampe KF, McCann MA. *AMA Handbook of Poisonous and Injurious Plants.* Chicago, IL: American Medical Association; 1985

Ogzewalla CD, Bonfiglio JF, Sigell LT. Common plants and their toxicity. *Pediatr Clin North Am.* 1987;34:1557-1598

Spoerke D, Evans B, Linaburg B. *The Hidden Hazards in House and Garden Plants.* Missoula, MT: Pictorial Histories Publishing Company Inc; 1991

Snakebite

Available Forms and Sources: Poisonous snakes bite an estimated 8000 people annually in the United States and about 12 to 15 fatalities are recorded each year. Approximately 20 species of poisonous snakes are found naturally in the United States and include pit vipers that have fangs, such as rattlesnakes, cottonmouths (water moccasins), and copperheads, and coral snakes that inject venom through fixed teeth in a chewing motion. At least 20% of bites by pit vipers are "dry" with no venom injected.

Children are at relatively greater risk for severe pit viper envenomation because the "pits," or heat receptors between the eyes and nostrils of the snake, more accurately sense the size, or heat mass, of a small child as compared to larger adults, resulting in a full discharge of a larger dose of venom.

Mechanism of Toxicity: Pit viper venoms are complex mixtures of proteins with enzymatic activity. These enzymes are capable of causing injury to most organ systems. Coral snake venom is primarily a neurotoxin affecting both the central and peripheral nervous systems.

Toxic Dose: The primary variables in snakebites are the amount of venom injected by the snake and the particular species involved. An adult pit viper or coral snake that has not recently released stored venom can deliver a potentially lethal dose to an adult or child. Snakes are capable of envenomation at birth. There is a wide range in toxicity among North American pit viper venoms, with the Mojave rattlesnake being the most toxic and the copperhead the least toxic.

Signs and Symptoms: Pit viper envenomations almost always produce local pain, ecchymosis, and ascending swelling. In addition fasciculations and paresthesias may be noted. Systemic signs include coagulation disorders, thrombocytopenia, hypotension, respiratory paralysis, pulmonary edema, and renal dysfunction. Coral snake envenomation produces light-headedness, weakness, tremors, nausea, vomiting, and cranial nerve dysfunction with respiratory insufficiency.

Diagnostic Testing: There is no readily available laboratory test to confirm a suspected snakebite. Diagnosis must be based on the history and clinical presentation of the patient.

General Treatment: If an envenomation has occurred, the patient should be observed closely and monitored in the hospital for at least 24 hours with supportive care and laboratory monitoring. Administration of antivenin is advised if a coral snake envenomation has occurred or is suspected, even if the patient is asymptomatic.

Antidote: A polyvalent Crotalidae antivenin is available for the treatment of envenomation by the copperhead, water moccasin, and all species of rattlesnakes (see Table 2, p 16, for specific dosing). This product is produced from horse serum and is potentially allergenic. It is rarely needed for copperhead bites. Its use for bites from other species should be limited to situations in which significant symptoms are present or likely to occur (ie, hypotension, bleeding, or threat of vascular compromise to a limb). Skin testing for allergic reactions is recommended prior to use but should not be performed unless a decision has been made to use antivenin because skin testing alone may sensitize the patient to the horse serum.

When antivenin is indicated usually a minimum of 5 vials is necessary for the first dose. Subsequent doses may be titrated, often in 5-vial increments. The end point of therapy is when further deterioration stops, improvement in perfusion is seen, or shock is diminished. Usually 5 to 15 vials of antivenin are needed. Up to 40 vials have been used following severe envenomations.

North American coral snake antivenin is commercially available for bites from the Eastern or Texas coral snake. There is no effective antivenin for the Sonoran (Arizona) coral snake. Antivenin should be given even if the patient is asymptomatic whenever envenomation is suspected. This antivenin is made from horse serum and may produce allergic symptoms. The patient should undergo skin testing for prior sensitization. The usual starting dose is 3 to 5 vials. The dose can be repeated if symptoms develop or persist.

Specific Treatment: Snakebites are contaminated wounds and require meticulous cleansing. Tetanus prophylaxis should be given if necessary. Prophylaxis with broad-spectrum antibiotics should be given to patients exposed to significant envenomation or those who are debilitated. Most envenomations occur on extremities. For pit viper envenomation, slight elevation of extremities helps control swelling. The wound site should be warm-packed to help ease the pain.

Cold packs and tourniquets should not be used because they have been shown to increase regional tissue damage. Incision and drainage of the wound are not generally recommended, although data from animal studies suggest that some venom can be removed if the procedure is performed within minutes of the envenomation. Fasciotomy is rarely necessary because swelling is usually superficial, and should be reserved for cases in which objective evidence demonstrates compromised blood flow.

Patient Monitoring: Patients with pit viper bites should be carefully monitored for at least 4 to 8 hours in an emergency facility for the development of symptoms. Symptomatic patients should be monitored in the hospital for at least 24 hours with serial monitoring of coagulation studies and limb perfusion. The later can be monitored with Doppler pulses, a pulse oximeter attached to a digit, or by capillary refill.

Patients with coral snakebite envenomation should be monitored in the hospital for 24 to 48 hours with serial neurological checks.

Enhanced Elimination: Enhanced elimination techniques are of no proven value.

References

Curry SC, Kraner JC, Kunkel DB, Ryan PJ, et al. Noninvasive vascular studies in management of rattlesnake envenomations to extremities. *Ann Emerg Med.* 1985;14:1081-1084

Gold BS, Barish RA. Venomous snakebites: current concepts in diagnosis, treatment, and management. *Emerg Med Clin North Am.* 1992;10:249-267

Russell FE. Snake venom poisoning. *Vet Hum Toxicol.* 1991;33:584-586

Treatment of snakebite in the USA. *Med Lett Drugs Ther.* 1982;24:87-89

Spider Bites

Available Forms and Sources: Almost all North American spiders produce venom. It is estimated that fewer than 50 of the more than 20 000 species, however, are capable of envenomating humans. Two species of spiders are of particular concern and are included in this discussion—*Latrodectus* species (widow spider) and *Loxosceles* species (brown recluse spiders). Other species such as *Phidippus*, or jumping spider; *Chiracanthium*, or running spider; *Lycosa,* or wolf spider; and *Argiope,* or orb weaver may produce necrotic lesions similar to the *Loxosceles* species but are less common and will not be considered separately.

Mechanism of Toxicity: The venom produced by widow spiders contains an extremely potent neurotoxin that causes the rapid release of several endogenous neurotransmitters from presynaptic nerve membranes. The venom from the brown recluse spider contains several tissue destructive enzymes capable of producing local injury and allowing the spread of venom. It is believed that the tissue necrosis that develops, however, is primarily the result of liposomes released by polymorphonuclear cells attracted to the area of the bite. Venom components may also cause lysis of red blood cells.

Toxic Dose: The venom from one bite of either species is capable of producing significant symptoms in an adult. Children are more susceptible to the toxic effects of *Latrodectus* venom probably because they receive a larger dose of venom per body weight.

Signs and Symptoms: Bites from widow spiders cause pain and muscle spasm in the bitten limb. The bite may not be immediately painful, and local inflammatory symptoms are mild or absent. Pain begins in the regional lymph nodes and quickly spreads to muscles producing spasm, chest pain, or abdominal cramping that may be confused with acute appendicitis. Pain may be quite severe and may be associated with hypertension and tachypnea. Symptoms usually peak within a few hours of the envenomation and subside over a period of hours to days. Death is rare.

Bites from brown recluse spiders are usually painless, with the victim unaware of the bite until local symptoms develop. Typical lesions develop within a few hours with a central bleb surrounded by concentric rings of pale ischemic tissue and erythema. Most envenomations probably do not progress any further and resolve without complications. In some cases, the bleb slowly enlarges and turns purple to black over a few days. Breakdown of the bleb may lead to a central ulcer that heals very slowly over several weeks. Necrotic areas may become large and sometimes require skin grafting. A systemic reaction (loxoscelism) occurs in a few cases characterized by fever, chills, nausea, myelagia, and hemolysis that may be accompanied by disseminated intravascular coagulation (DIC), renal failure, and seizures. Systemic symptoms may progress over a period of several days after envenomation.

Diagnostic Testing: Diagnosis is based on the clinical presentation and evidence of envenomation. No specific diagnostic test is available. Favorable response to the administration of *Latro-*

dectus antivenin has been used as a diagnostic test to rule out other serious abdominal processes.

General Treatment: Bite sites should be thoroughly cleaned and tetanus prophylaxis administered as necessary. Acute symptoms associated with widow spider envenomation usually require hospital evaluation with possible admission for the control of pain and muscle spasm. Brown recluse envenomation can usually be treated on an outpatient basis unless systemic symptoms develop or severe necrosis requires wound care or skin grafting.

Antidote: *Latrodectus* (widow spider) antivenin (**see Table 2, p 16, for specific dosing**) is commercially available and can be used if symptoms warrant. The antivenin is equine in origin and is associated with serum sickness and a risk of anaphylaxis. It should be reserved for either severe cases or cases of severe abdominal pain when it is important to distinguish envenomation from other operable abdominal conditions. If the antivenin is used, skin testing is recommended prior to administration.

Specific Treatment: Muscle spasms from widow spider bites can generally be treated with either intravenous calcium gluconate (0.2 mL/kg to a maximum of 10 mL) or intravenous methocarbamol (Robaxin) (**see Table 3, p 22, for specific dosing**). Repeat doses as necessary to control pain. Diazepam has been used but has proven to be less effective than calcium or methocarbamol. One study has described the successful use of intravenous dantrolene.

The treatment of brown recluse bites is very controversial. Good general wound care and the use of antipruritic agents should be emphasized. Excision of the bite early after it has occurred, while favored by some, has not been shown to improve outcome and is clearly unnecessary for most bites, which will resolve without complications. Steroids are also of no proven value. Limited data in humans have suggested the use of dapsone, an agent that inhibits leukocyte migration. The dose is 0.5 mg/kg/d for 2 days increasing to 1 mg/kg/d if tolerated; continue therapy until the lesion resolves. Side effects from dapsone include methemoglobinemia and hemolytic anemia (particularly in patients with G6PD deficiency) and it should be used with caution and monitoring. Further data are needed before it can be routinely recommended. One study has reported good results with the use of hyperbaric oxygen in a small group of patients.

Patient Monitoring: Patients experiencing brown recluse bites should be closely followed for the development of systemic toxicity including hemoglobinuria. Monitor the patient for secondary infection, although it is not common.

Enhanced Elimination: Enhanced elimination techniques are of no proven value.

References

Alario A, Price G, Stahl R, et al. Cutaneous necrosis following spider bite: a case report and review. *Pediatrics*. 1987;79:618-621

King LE, Rees RS. Dapsone treatment of a brown recluse bite. *JAMA*. 1983; 250:648

Rees RS, Altenbern P, Lynch J, King LE. Brown recluse spider bites: a comparison of early surgical excision versus dapsone and delayed surgical excision. *Ann Surg*. 1985;202:659-663

Vorse H, Seccareccio P, Woodruff K, et al. Disseminated intravascular coagulopathy following fatal brown recluse spider bite (necrotic arachnidism). *J Pediatr*. 1972;80:1035-1037

FOREIGN BODIES INCLUDING BUTTON BATTERIES

Available Forms and Sources: Foreign bodies commonly lodge in either the gastrointestinal tract or respiratory tract; over 75% occur in children younger than 6 years. The variety of foreign bodies includes coins, safety pins (open and closed), nails, screws, buttons, button batteries, and small toys. Coins are the most common foreign body ingested by children. Some foods such as nuts, raisins, seeds, hard candy, sausage-shaped meats and raw carrots are likely to be aspirated and become foreign bodies in the respiratory tract. Aspiration of foreign bodies may be facilitated by drugs and alcohol intoxication, seizures, anesthesia, or head trauma that reduce the conscious state and diminish the airway protective reflexes.

Ingestion of button batteries is becoming more frequent and presents some unique problems. Button disc batteries are marked with imprint codes that allow identification of the manufacturer and the contents. The components of batteries vary as follows: calculator-type batteries contain mercury and silver oxides, camera batteries contain mercury and manganese oxides, hand-held computer game batteries contain mercury and silver oxides, hearing aid batteries contain mercury, silver oxides or zinc, and watch batteries contain silver, mercury or manganese oxides, and lithium. An alkali battery usually contains 26% to 45% sodium or potassium hydroxide. Hearing aid button batteries are the most common type ingested.

Mechanism of Toxicity: The major mechanism of injury with foreign bodies is from mechanical obstruction. Laryngotracheal airway obstruction may result in hypoxic damage. Bronchial obstruction may result in pneumonia and atelectasis. Esophageal obstruction may result in perforation and fistulae. Obstruction in the gastrointestinal tract may result in perforation and peritonitis.

Most foreign bodies are not systemically toxic, although in one case lead toxicity and death were caused by a retained curtain weight. Button batteries that range in diameter from 7.9 to 25 mm may open and release their contents. Complications, however, occur in less than 2% of button battery ingestions and are more likely to be associated with the ingestion of the larger sized lithium batteries. The mechanism of injury is related to leakage of the alkali or electrolytes, electrolysis, and pressure necrosis. Mercuric oxide released from button batteries in the gastrointestinal tract is converted into elemental mercury, which is poorly absorbed and rarely produces toxicity. Mercuric oxide cells are reported to be more likely to fragment than other types of button batteries.

Signs and Symptoms: The manifestations depend on the nature, size, configuration, location, and time the foreign body remains at one site. Most foreign body ingestions are asymptomatic.

Respiratory tract foreign bodies. Laryngotracheal obstruction may be life-threatening, affect breathing, and cause dramatic symptoms including stridor, dysphonia, retractions, cyanosis, and diminished air exchange on auscultation. Round objects can completely obstruct the airway. Facial petechiae may develop secondary to increased intrathoracic pressure.

Bronchial foreign bodies cause air trapping, coughing, wheezing, and cyanosis. Unilateral wheezing in a child, wheezing in a child that responds poorly to routine asthma therapy, or deterioration of a child's condition despite appropriate medical therapy should indicate the possibility of aspiration of a foreign body. Pneumonia and atelectasis are commonly present.

Esophageal foreign bodies. Foreign bodies in the esophagus are most likely to be located at the three areas of physiologic narrowing—the level of the thoracic inlet, the arch of the aorta indentation, and the cardioesophageal sphincter. Up to 30% of children with coins in the esophagus are asymptomatic. Others may have manifestations that include refusal to eat, dysphagia, excess salivation, gagging, vomiting, throat and neck pain, the sensation of a foreign body, or substernal discomfort.

The complications of a coin impacted in the esophagus include asymptomatic perforation of the esophagus, tracheoesophageal fistula, esophageal-aortic fistula, and airway obstruction. Respiratory obstructive symptoms from esophageal foreign bodies are due to compression of the posterior tracheal wall by a firm mass high in the esophagus. This is more likely with large coins or button batteries.

Gastrointestinal tract foreign bodies. Over 95% of swallowed foreign bodies reaching the stomach pass through the gastrointestinal tract without incident although sharp pointed objects and long objects may lodge in the wall and cause perforation. Long foreign bodies in a young child or infant may not be able to pass through the duodenal C loop or may become lodged at the ligament of Treitz, in a Meckel's diverticulum, or at the ileocecal valve.

Diagnostic Testing: Radiography is especially important in symptomatic patients, even if the symptoms are transient; in patients who ingest quarter-sized foreign bodies or larger; and in patients with prior esophageal surgery or strictures. A frontal view of the chest and a lateral neck view should be obtained. If the foreign body is not localized, an abdominal roentgenogram is optional because foreign bodies that have moved beyond the esophagus are rarely of clinical concern.

The search for nonradiopaque foreign bodies (wood, buttons, glass marbles, bone fragments, aluminum pull tabs, or plastic) may include a soft-tissue lateral neck roentgenogram, a posteroanterior view of the oropharynx and neck, inspiratory and expiratory chest roentgenograms, and/or a lateral decubitus roentgenogram of the chest. Consider fluoroscopy when the patient is unable to cooperate or there are equivocal findings on the chest roentgenogram. A contrast esophagram study with dilute barium may be helpful to outline the nonradiopaque object. If these procedures fail to reveal the foreign body, endoscopy should be considered. Although usually unnecessary, in certain cases a dilute barium swallow examination may be performed 24 to 36 hours after removal of the foreign body to exclude a fistula.

Controversy exists over whether all children who swallow coins should undergo roentgenographic examination. Most recent studies, however, advocate obtaining a radiograph in a child who ingests a coin, since many esophageal foreign bodies are asymptomatic. On anteroposterior chest roentgenograms, coins orient themselves in the esophagus in the frontal or coronal plane with the full circle wide diameter, or "on face." A coin in the trachea has its axis in the sagittal plane with the wide diameter "on end."

The use of a metal detector has been successful in locating coins ingested by children. This technique identified the presence or absence of coins correctly in 93% of patients.

General Treatment: The management must be individualized and depends on the clinical condition of the patient and the nature, size, configuration, location, and duration of the foreign body at the site. There are few reports of successful expulsion of foreign bodies after the administration of syrup of ipecac and it is not recommended.

Laryngotracheobronchial foreign bodies. These objects should be removed by immediate laryngotracheobronchoscopy under general endotracheal anesthesia with good control of the airway. If no foreign body is found, esophagoscopy should be performed to exclude the possibility of a mass in the esophagus pressing on the posterior wall of the trachea.

Esophageal foreign bodies. These foreign bodies require urgent but not emergent endoscopic removal. Early removal is indicated when there are noteworthy symptoms because of the hazard of obstruction, aspiration, or erosion of the thin esophageal wall. Removal should be performed immediately if the patient is unable to handle secretions, if the foreign body is in the upper third of the esophagus, or if it is sharp. Foreign bodies in the esophagus should not be allowed to remain there more than 24 hours. Patients with esophageal disorders such as strictures secondary to tracheoesophageal fistulae repair are prone to having foreign bodies lodge in the esophagus, and prompt removal is necessary.

The methods of removal include observation for 12 to 24 hours for spontaneous passage, endoscopy, Foley catheter, and bougienage. The best method of removal of foreign bodies is still controversial. A recent study of 57 children concluded all but one could be treated using a Foley balloon technique or the esophageal bougie technique. The method of removal depends entirely on the experience and preference of the surgeon or the specialist. Endoscopy is accomplished under endotracheal anesthesia to establish good control of the airway and avoid aspiration. In some cases the anesthesia given for endoscopy will produce enough relaxation to allow the foreign body to pass into the stomach. Always obtain an roentgenogram immediately before endoscopy to insure that the radiopaque foreign body is still in the esophagus.

The Foley catheter technique is used to remove smooth foreign bodies such as coins from the esophagus and is reserved for patients who are sufficiently awake to retain good airway protective reflexes. This method of removal should be performed by those skilled in its use and prepared to deal with all possible complications including aspiration of the foreign body. It is not recommended if the foreign object has been present for over 24 hours or if it is sharp or pointed. Some of the advocates of this technique have recently recommended against its use for removal of button batteries.

Esophageal bougienage must be performed within 24 hours of ingestion of the foreign body with the position of the object confirmed by roentgenogram. The technique involves the passage of a well-lubricated, round-tipped, weighted bougie dilator from the oropharynx through the esophagus to the stomach with the patient sitting upright. The physician rolls the foreign body, usually a coin, into the stomach.

Coins lodged in the esophagus usually pass into the stomach within the first few hours. The removal of the coin depends on the location (upper esophageal lodgement is more emergent), the time that has passed since ingestion (foreign bodies should be removed within 24 hours), prior clinical condition of the patient, and the experience of the physician. For impacted meat in the upper two thirds of the esophagus, emergency endoscopic removal is recommended. The use of papain enzyme digestion (meat tenderizer) is not recommended because it has been associated with hypernatremia and digestive erosions of the esophagus.

Glucagon has been used successfully in some cases to relax the esophagus and allow the foreign body to pass into the stomach.

Gastrointestinal foreign bodies. Almost all foreign bodies in the stomach and intestines will pass through the tract without assistance. Rounded or cuboid objects rarely cause symptoms once they reach the stomach. Over 95% of gastrointestinal foreign bodies navigate the entire tract without symptoms or the need of therapy. In asymptomatic patients with a smooth-blunt gastric foreign body, the average transit time for the object to be passed in the stool was <72 hours in 85% of patients, by 7 days in 95% of patients, and by 2 weeks in 99% of patients. Although not necessary for most ingestions, stools may be examined for the foreign body. A useful method is to drape cheesecloth over the toilet bowl under the seat and wash away the stool with hot water. A repeated roentgenogram of the abdomen may be considered 7 days after ingestion if examination of the stools fails to detect the foreign body.

Long thin or sharp pointed objects may lodge in the intestinal wall and cause perforation and peritonitis. Hat pins are particularly dangerous. Surgery should be considered if there are signs of peritonitis or a sharp object remains stationary for prolonged periods. The development of fever, vomiting, hematemesis, or melena in any patient with a known foreign body ingestion requires immediate surgical evaluation.

The use of a magnet attached to an orogastric tube passed into the stomach for metallic foreign bodies has been successful. There is, however, a danger of aspiration.

Specific treatment for button batteries. Contact a poison center to identify the ingredients in the battery. If the battery is in the esophagus or respiratory tract, immediate endoscopic removal is indicated. The "Foley catheter technique" should not be used because batteries lodged in the esophagus have a high rate of producing local damage.

If the battery has passed beyond the esophagus, do not attempt initial endoscopic removal because the failure rate is 70% and most will pass without difficulty. The patient may be sent home to be observed for vomiting, tarry or bloody stools, or abdominal pain. All stools should be strained to retrieve the battery. Asymptomatic patients may receive a cathartic. If the patient remains asymptomatic, follow-up roentgenograms once or twice a week should be considered. If the battery does not pass the pylorus within 48 hours it is unlikely to pass. These patients may benefit from an attempt at endoscopic retrieval. Lack of movement of the battery is not an indication for immediate surgical intervention but surgical consultation is advised at this time. If the battery appears lodged in a Meckel's diverticulum or if peritoneal irritation occurs, surgical removal is indicated.

If a mercury disc battery opens, it is not necessary to monitor concentrations of the mercury, unless there are manifestations of toxicity. Mercury levels and chelation therapy should be reserved for those patients who develop signs of mercury toxicity.

Batteries lodged in the auditory canal, nose, or other orifices should be removed immediately. A magnetic screwdriver may aid in removal.

References

Bonadio WA. Coin ingestion: small change, big problem. *Contemp Pediatr.* 1992;9:71-88

Bonadio WA, Jona JZ, Glicklich M, Cohen R. Esophageal bougienage technique for coin ingestion in children. *J Pediatr Surg.* 1988;23:917-918

Foster DL. Pediatric coin ingestions. *AJDC.* 1990;144:450-452

Hawkins DB. Removal of blunt foreign bodies from the esophagus. *Ann Otol Rhinol Laryngol.* 1990;99:935-940

Hodge D, Tecklenburg F, Fleisher G. Coin ingestion: does every child need a radiograph? *Ann Emerg Med.* 1985;14:443-446

Kelly JE, Leech MH, Carr MG. A safe and cost-effective protocol for the management of esophageal coins in children. *J Pediatr Surg.* 1993;28:898-900

Litovitz T, Schmitz BF. Ingestion of cylindrical and button batteries: an analysis of 2382 cases. *Pediatrics.* 1992;89:747-757

Shunk JE, Corneli H, Bolte R. Pediatric coin ingestions: a prospective study of coin location and symptoms. *AJDC.* 1989;143:546-54

Stringer MD, Capps SN. Rationalizing the management of swallowed coins in children. *Br Med J.* 1991;302:1321-1322

INDEX

Page numbers in boldface type indicate the page on which a major discussion of the entry can be found; pages with a *t* indicate tabular material.